T0131061

The

FUTURE OF FENTANYL
and OTHER SYNTHETIC OPIOIDS

Bryce Pardo, Jirka Taylor, Jonathan P. Caulkins, Beau Kilmer,
Peter Reuter, Bradley D. Stein

For more information on this publication, visit www.rand.org/t/RR3117

Library of Congress Cataloging-in-Publication Data is available for this publication.
ISBN: 978-1-9774-0338-4

Published by the RAND Corporation, Santa Monica, Calif.
© Copyright 2019 RAND Corporation
RAND® is a registered trademark.

Cover: Fentanyl molecule structure/serge01/Adobe Stock.

www.rand.org

This report is dedicated to Mark A. R. Kleiman, our friend, colleague, and inspiration. As this analysis describes, the fentanyl problem is unlike any preceding drug epidemic in fundamental and challenging ways. Likewise, Mark was unlike any other who labored in the field of drug policy. He was a one-of-a-kind thinker who challenged status quo beliefs by grappling with the fundamental behaviors of people and markets—always with the determination to make the world a better place, just as he has made each of us better scholars and better people through his wise mentoring. Mark will be long remembered by the field and missed by us all.

Mark A. R. Kleiman
1951–2019

Preface

The U.S. opioid crisis worsened dramatically with the arrival of synthetic opioids, such as fentanyl, which are now responsible for tens of thousands of deaths annually. This crisis is far-reaching and even with prompt, targeted responses, many of the problems will persist for decades to come. RAND Corporation researchers have completed numerous opioid-related projects and have more underway for such clients and grantors as the Agency for Healthcare Research and Quality, the Assistant Secretary of Health and Human Services for Planning and Evaluation, the National Institute on Drug Abuse, the White House Office of National Drug Control Policy, and Pew Charitable Trusts. Researchers have advanced an understanding of the dimensions of the problem, some of the causes and consequences, and the effectiveness of different responses. However, no one has yet addressed the full scope of the problems associated with opioid use disorder and overdose deaths.

Beginning in late 2018, the RAND Corporation initiated a comprehensive effort to understand the problem and responses to help reverse the tide of the opioid crisis. The project involves dozens of RAND experts in a variety of areas, including drug policy, substance use treatment, health care, public health, criminal justice, child welfare and other social services, education, and employment. In this work, we intend to describe the entire opioid ecosystem, identifying the components of the system and how they interact; establish concepts of success and metrics to gauge progress; and construct a simulation model of large parts of the ecosystem to permit an evaluation of the full effects of policy responses. We dedicated project resources and communications expertise to ensure that our products and dissemination activities are optimized for reaching our primary intended audiences: policymakers and other critical decisionmakers and influencers, including those in the public, private, and nonprofit sectors. The project is ambitious in scope and will not be the last word on the subject, but by tackling the crisis in a comprehensive fashion, it promises to offer a unique and broad perspective in terms of the way the nation understands and responds to this urgent national problem.

Ten years ago, few would have predicted that illicitly manufactured synthetic opioids from overseas would sweep through parts of Appalachia, New England, and the Midwest. As drug markets are flooded by fentanyl and other synthetic opioids, policymakers, researchers, and the public are trying to understand what to make of it and how to respond. The synthesis of heroin in the late 19th century displaced morphine and forever changed the opiate landscape, and we might again be standing at the precipice of a new era. Cheap, accessible, and mass-produced synthetic opioids could very well displace heroin, generating important and hard-to-predict consequences.

As part of RAND's project to stem the tide of the opioid crisis, this mixed-methods report offers a systematic assessment of the past, present, and possible futures of fentanyl and other synthetic opioids found in illicit drug markets in the United States. This research is rooted in secondary data analysis, literature and document reviews, international case studies, and key informant interviews. Our goal is to provide local, state, and national decisionmakers who are concerned about rising overdose trends with insights that might improve their understanding of and responses to this problem. We also hope to provide new information to other researchers, media sources, and the public, who are contributing to these critical policy discussions.

RAND Ventures

The RAND Corporation is a research organization that develops solutions to public policy challenges to help make communities throughout the world safer and more secure, healthier and more prosperous. RAND is nonprofit, nonpartisan, and committed to the public interest.

RAND Ventures is a vehicle for investing in policy solutions. Philanthropic contributions support our ability to take the long view, tackle tough and often-controversial topics, and share our findings in innovative and compelling ways. RAND's research findings and recommendations are based on data and evidence, and therefore do not necessarily reflect the policy preferences or interests of its clients, donors, or supporters.

Funding for this venture was provided by gifts from RAND supporters and income from operations.

Contents

Figures

Tables

Summary

The number of opioid-related deaths in the United States is truly astounding. There were on the order of 50,000 opioid-involved overdose fatalities in 2018, which is roughly similar to the magnitude of deaths from HIV/AIDS at its peak in 1995 (Centers for Disease Control and Prevention, 2013; Ruhm, 2018; Ahmad et al., 2019). The rates of overdose fatalities involving heroin or other semisynthetic or natural opioids (which are mostly prescription drugs; see Appendix A for terms) have slowed in recent years and are now outnumbered two to one by overdoses involving synthetic opioids. Ciccarone (2017, p. 107) refers to a "triple wave epidemic:" The first wave was prescription opioids, the second wave was heroin, and the third—and ongoing—wave is synthetic opioids.

There are many different synthetic opioids, but analyses of death certificate records show that most synthetic opioid overdoses as of 2016 involve fentanyl (Hedegaard et al., 2018; Spencer et al., 2019). Similarly, drug seizure databases indicate a sharp rise in the number of exhibits containing fentanyl, from slightly fewer than 1,000 in 2013 to more than 59,000 in 2017 (U.S. Drug Enforcement Administration, 2018e), although some of that increase might be a function of greater law enforcement efforts aimed at detecting and seizing fentanyl and other synthetic opioids.

Ten years ago, few would have predicted that illicitly manufactured fentanyl from overseas would sweep through British Columbia or parts of Appalachia and New England. As drug markets are flooded with extremely potent opioids, policymakers, researchers, and the public are trying to understand what to make of it and how to respond. Much as the synthesis of heroin in the late 19th century displaced morphine and forever changed the opiate landscape, the country may again be standing at the precipice of a new era: Inexpensive, accessible, and mass-produced synthetic opioids might displace heroin, which could have important and hard-to-predict consequences.

This mixed-methods report offers a systematic assessment of the past, present, and possible futures of fentanyl and other synthetic opioids found in illicit drug markets in the United States. This report is rooted in secondary data analysis, literature and document reviews, international case studies, and key informant interviews. Our goal is to provide local, state, and national decisionmakers with insights and analyses that might improve their understanding of and responses to the problem of rising overdoses and transitioning markets. We also hope to provide new information to researchers, media sources, and the public, who are contributing to these critical policy discussions.

Fentanyl and Other Synthetic Opioids Are Becoming Dominant in Some Parts of the United States and Canada, but Remain Less Common in Other Parts of These Countries

Our analysis shows that synthetic opioid overdoses increased dramatically between 2013 and 2017 but remained concentrated regionally, notably in Appalachia, the Midatlantic, and New England in the United States and in Alberta, British Columbia, and Ontario in Canada. There is considerable spatial overlap in rising overdoses and seizure exhibit counts in the same parts of the United States. Furthermore, some U.S. markets are experiencing *declines* in seizures and fatal overdoses involving heroin—especially for heroin overdoses that did not involve synthetic opioids. This suggests that, in some markets, fentanyl is replacing—not just adulterating or supplementing—heroin, a trend that also is reported in parts of Canada.

At the same time, some markets appear to be diversifying from fentanyl to a broader variety of new synthetic opioids. For instance,

Ohio reported a large number of seizures containing carfentanil, which is much more potent than fentanyl and was a contributing factor to the many overdoses in that state in 2017. Product variation could exacerbate harms; users and dealers might not know the strength or effects of new drugs. Our analysis of seizures across other states shows variation in supply, with some states dominated by a single synthetic opioid—fentanyl—while others report a variety of chemicals (see Chapter Two).

A Confluence of Factors, Including the Dissemination of Simplified and Novel Synthesis Methods and Increased E-Commerce, Helps Explain the Surge in Synthetic Opioids

Illicitly manufactured synthetic opioids have entered U.S. drug markets several times since the late 1970s, but these early outbreaks were generally localized and short-lived (see Table S.1). Given that fentanyl is cheaper and more potent than heroin, some experts predicted long

Table S.1
Comparing Aspects of U.S. Fentanyl Outbreaks

Aspect	Previous Outbreaks	Today's Outbreak
Location	Generally localized	Not localized, although there is regional variation
Duration	Generally short; only one lasted more than two years	Nearly six years
Chemicals	Fewer analogs; no reports of super-potent opioids (e.g., carfentanil)	Fentanyl dominates, but there are many analogs and super-potent opioids
Source	Often labs in the United States, with one exception	Almost all is imported, mostly from China and Mexico
Distribution	Limited, although two employed traditional illicit market actors	More widespread; both traditional illicit market actors and mail or internet order
Sold as	Often heroin, although some noted it showing up in cocaine	Heroin and prescription pills, but an increasing share of cocaine and psychostimulant overdoses mention synthetic opioids

ago that it would eclipse heroin, yet this has only recently become a significant problem. Why?

Some speculate that shocks to the heroin supply might have contributed to fentanyl's rise in the United States; indeed, that appears to have been a factor in Estonia 20 years ago. We are skeptical that this factor alone explains the spread of synthetic opioids, given that, more recently, fentanyl has simultaneously appeared in Canada and parts of Europe that have not experienced heroin supply shocks. Furthermore, there is disagreement about the direction of the recent trend in the purity-adjusted retail price for heroin in the United States, which raises questions about the degree to which a heroin supply shock occurred (see Appendix B for more information on price trends).

Rather than pointing to an increased demand for opioids or possible heroin supply shocks, a confluence of supply-side factors likely helps explain fentanyl's rise since 2013. One factor is that, during earlier outbreaks in the United States, production was limited to a few capable chemists, and bottlenecks in production and/or distribution slowed fentanyl's diffusion. Law enforcement was able to detect and shut down production before it spread to multiple sources. That strategy faces challenges in the contemporary era because production is based in China or Mexico, not in the United States. China's economy has grown at levels that outpace regulatory oversight (particularly its pharmaceutical and chemical industries), allowing suppliers to avoid regulatory scrutiny and U.S. law enforcement (O'Connor, 2017; Pardo, 2018).

Another factor is that fentanyl and other synthetic opioids are well-suited for the internet age. The rediscovery and manufacture of these chemicals has been aided by the online dissemination of novel, easier, and more-efficient synthesis methods.

Traditional drug trafficking organizations play a role in fentanyl distribution, but so do e-commerce and online shopping. Fentanyl's potency is such that a small quantity can be easily shipped directly to buyers halfway around the world for a modest fee.

International package delivery existed in the 20th century, but innovations that enhance online privacy (e.g., BitCoin, anonymous browsing) aid online trade in contraband. These operational shifts have expanded the once-limited distribution networks, making synthetic opioids accessible to anyone with an internet connection and a mailing address, thereby connecting low-level wholesale dealers to international producers in ways that bypass traditional drug distribution networks.

Much Can Be Learned From Other Countries' Experiences with Synthetic Opioids

Problems generated by synthetic opioids are not unique to North America; thus, there is much to be gained from examining the drug markets of other countries, a few of which have seen fentanyl become dominant in their illicit opioid markets or have experienced other notable market disruptions. Indicators of interest include the extent of fentanyl mixed with heroin, the availability of fentanyl analogs, and the timing of market changes. This international variation is not dissimilar from differences observed among individual U.S. states, some of which have been dominated by fentanyl (New Hampshire), by fentanyl analogs (Ohio), by a mix of fentanyl and heroin (Kentucky), or mostly by heroin (California). Therefore, just as we show variability across international jurisdictions, there is also variability across states in the United States. It would be inaccurate to speak of a homogeneous U.S. synthetic opioid problem.

Canada's experience with synthetic opioids is similar to that of the United States in timing, trajectory, and severity, perhaps in part because of the existence of a prior prescription opioid crisis in both countries. Consequently, the Canadian response could offer relevant lessons for the United States, although there are notable differences in the delivery of public health and social services in both countries.

In contrast, the European experience is limited to a handful of small countries with decreasing opioid use and with relatively few new users entering markets. In addition, while the nonprescribed use of prescription opioids—in particular, tramadol—has been a concern in some European countries, the extent of this problem has not been comparable with the situation in North America.

The European experiences might offer insights into potential future issues and trends. Estonia hosts arguably the world's only long-standing, mature fentanyl market, and so can offer one window into the future. Latvia, although it is adjacent to Estonia, provides another view. Its market skipped the fentanyl phase and proceeded directly to fentanyl analogs, which are sometimes more powerful. The available data suggest that this pattern has not been seen in any North American jurisdiction so far. Notably, this transition has failed to produce permanent increases in drug-related deaths in Latvia. Thus, if the mortality data are correct, Latvia's experience suggests that domination by synthetic opioids does not automatically result in much higher death rates. Sweden demonstrates the possibility of having an illicit fentanyl market that features a novel product (e.g., nasal spray), is separate from the heroin market, and has distinct modes of distribution and marketing (e.g., fentanyl sold as analogs online to end users). Sweden's experience also points to the possibility of substantially disrupting distribution networks, as exemplified by successful law enforcement operations in the country.

Supplier Decisions, Not User Demand, Drive the Transition to Fentanyl

The history of drug use and drug problems has been marked by a sequence of epidemics, but the synthetic opioid problem is different. Whereas previous epidemics often were spurred by growing demand, the transition to fentanyl and other synthetic opioids appears to be a supplier-led phenomenon. To date, it also primarily involves an adulterant, not the drug that most users seek out by name. Thus, synthetic opioids are best thought of as a new strategic device for dealers seeking to lower costs or skirt drug control laws, not as a newly popular drug among users (although, over time, individuals in some markets might become accustomed to fentanyl and seek it out).

To elaborate, most drug epidemics begin with a rapid—even "contagious"—spread of initiation, primarily among youth, often amid ignorance, overconfidence, or naivete about the drug's risks. Over time, as some users escalate to frequent and/or chronic use, the reputation of the drug changes (Courtwright, 2009; Musto, 1999). Then, initiation ebbs, and society is left with a residual pool of chronic users whose use persists, sometimes for decades.

Almost none of that script pertains to fentanyl. Fentanyl and other synthetic opioids are not a drug of initiation for most individuals, at least in markets in the United States. Its use typically does not spread by word-of-mouth contact among users; it penetrates markets when suppliers embrace it. It appears that few opioid users are looking for fentanyl and other synthetic opioids specifically, at least initially; indeed, many longtime heroin users prefer not to use these substances, given their shorter duration, lethality, and unpredictability, although some come to prefer fentanyl because of its ability to overcome users' tolerance (Ciccarone, Ondocsin, and Mars, 2017; Mars, Ondocsin, and Ciccarone, 2018b). Thus, the traditional epidemic framework largely fails to capture the dynamics of the problem.

Fentanyl's Spread Is Episodically Fast and Has Ratchet-Like Persistence

Once fentanyl gains a foothold, it appears capable of sweeping through a market very quickly. In Chapter Two, we describe how, in just a few years, fentanyl practically supplanted heroin in many markets in New Hampshire. That said, we also note in Chapter Two that, in a large area of the western United States, death rates from synthetic opioids remain far lower than those in New England. Illegally manufactured fentanyl and other synthetic opioids are not totally absent from the western United States, but they remained a minor presence, at least through 2017, per mortality and drug seizure data.[1]

---

[1] That said, media reports and provisional data from authorities have noted a sharp increase in overdose fatalities or drug seizures involving fentanyl in major markets in the western United States. In 2018, San Francisco attributed nearly 60 overdoses to fentanyl, a sixfold increase since 2015 (Allday, 2019). In Phoenix, Arizona, the police crime laboratory also has seen a sharp rise in retail-level seizures of counterfeit oxycodone tablets that contain fentanyl; from 43 in 2017 to more than 340 in the first five months of 2019 (Crenshaw, 2019).

One possible explanation is that some illegal markets might require a certain minimum scale in order to operate efficiently. Below that scale, an illegal market struggles. Above that scale, the market is resilient to enforcement and other disruptions. Such a situation can lead two otherwise similar places to have very different rates of use (e.g., low in one market and high in another).

One could crudely divide the world into two types of areas: those already beset by fentanyl and other synthetic opioids and those fighting to delay that transition. The second group has reason to be vigilant. Although prompt action could extinguish nascent fires—as happened, for example, in the United States from 2005 to 2007—the window of opportunity is small and might be closing. Prior outbreaks could be attributed to a single supply source. That is not true today with the arrival of mass-produced and cheap imports.

Furthermore, we know of no instance in which fentanyl attained a dominant position in the marketplace and then lost that position to another less potent opioid. To date, fentanyl's spread appears to be a one-way ratchet.[2] The same can be said about drug markets transitioning from morphine to more-potent heroin more than 100 years ago.

Synthetic Opioids Drive Up Deaths Rather Than the Number of Users

In Chapter Four, we observe that injection drug use in Estonia peaked in the 1990s, *before* the arrival of fentanyl. Elsewhere in Europe, the emergence of fentanyl generally occurred against the backdrop of declining opioid user populations. Likewise, we have not come across evidence pointing to fentanyl increasing either initiation or chronic use in the United States or Canada. Although opioid-use disorder is far more common than it was 20 years ago, that growth primarily has come from prescription opioids rather than fentanyl, and it occurred before 2014, rather than in the past few years. Thus, it seems fair to

---

[2] By *one-way ratchet*, we mean that the spread of fentanyl only increases.

say that fentanyl brought a wave of greater death and not a rising tide of more users.

That this problem is so different suggests that the response will also need to be different. Traditional approaches aimed at drug epidemics focus on preventing initiation, raising prices, and increasing treatment to suppress demand, but these efforts will not immediately reduce overdose deaths in areas that are already drowning in synthetic opioids. In these areas, reducing deaths quickly will require having conversations about interventions intended to reduce the risk of drug overdose, some of which are still controversial in the United States (see, e.g., McGinty et al., 2018; Kilmer et al., 2019).

A focus on reducing deaths and nonfatal synthetic opioid poisonings does not mean that jurisdictions need to abandon traditional approaches. But the fact that fentanyl and other synthetic opioids have driven up death rates sharply in jurisdictions in Canada and the United States spanning the range of traditional approaches to drug policy makes clear that some nontraditional, outside-the-box thinking will be required.

Problems with Synthetic Opioids Are Likely to Worsen Before They Improve, and States West of the Mississippi River Must Remain Vigilant

One of the most important—and depressing—insights in this analysis is that however bad the synthetic opioid problem is now, it is likely to get worse before it gets better. In Chapter Two, we show that the United States's synthetic opioid problem is not yet truly national in scope. Some regions have been acutely affected; others have been spared to date, at least in relative terms, but authorities in such regions should not be complacent.

In 2017, ten states accounted for one-third of all mentions of synthetic opioid overdoses, despite making up a little more than one-tenth of the nation's population. Conversely, almost three in ten states report synthetic opioid overdose death rates that are one-quarter of the national average of nine per 100,000. The math is simple and distressing: If the rest of the country had a synthetic opioid–involved death rate of half of New England's in 2017, that would come to about 38,000 synthetic opioid–involved fatal overdoses.[3]

That potent synthetic opioids now appear in counterfeit prescription medications is another concern. Those misusing diverted prescription pain relievers or other medications could be at substantial risk of overdose, should they incorrectly assume that these fakes are of genuine origin. Pills also might appeal to individuals who do not inject drugs.

The problem could worsen in other ways as well. Currently, synthetic opioids appear in postmortems of about half of overdose deaths involving cocaine and about one-quarter of those involving psychostimulants, again with sharp regional variation. Some users knowingly ingest heroin along with cocaine (which is sometimes referred to as *speedballing*) or methamphetamine (sometimes referred to as *goofballing*; Szalavitz, 2019). Others ingest stimulants containing fentanyl already, although it is not clear whether dealers intentionally adulterate stimulants with fentanyl or if it is accidental cross-contamination (Cauchon, 2019; Daly, 2019). This is worrisome because stimulant-only users are not opioid-tolerant and are much more likely to succumb to a fatal overdose. If cocaine users on the West Coast or more methamphetamine users generally were exposed to synthetic opioids, death rates would increase. In 2019, authorities reported multiple overdoses in California from individuals consuming fentanyl thought to be cocaine (Armenian et al., 2019; Byik, 2019).

Furthermore, fentanyl is not the most potent or deadly of the synthetic opioids. In 2017, Ohio and British Columbia saw a surge in deaths associated with carfentanil. Carfentanil also was, until recently, the clearly dominant synthetic opioid in Latvia (see Chapter Four). At face value, carfentanil's potency could make it an attractive alternative

---

[3] Some states in New England have relatively robust addiction treatment services and generous public health systems, making this a worrisome statistic. In 2017, there were nearly 3,300 overdoses involving synthetic opioids in the six states in New England, which comes to a crude overdose death rate of 22 per 100,000 residents. Multiplying a fatality rate of 11 per 100,000 across the remaining 44 states and the District of Columbia would amount to just more than 34,000 fatal overdoses.

for dealers but dosing out this substance in precise microgram quantities is extremely difficult.

In Chapter Five, we offer multiple scenarios for the future of fentanyl and other synthetic opioids in the United States and the factors that could shape them. No one knows how this will play out, but it would be prudent to prepare for the problem to get worse before it gets better and for it to persist for the indefinite future, not to "flash and recede."

Improving Surveillance and Monitoring Is Crucial

Governments have a unique responsibility for funding data collection and monitoring of drug use, drug problems, and drug markets. On that score, the U.S. government has failed and failed badly (see Appendix C). Whereas once the United States boasted the world's best drug data infrastructure for supporting evidence-informed decisionmaking, it now lags behind. For example, many countries now test wastewater to monitor and track drug consumption trends (Castiglioni, 2016). The United States has not made this a priority.

The HIV/AIDS crisis prompted large-scale investments in new data and monitoring systems, such as the National HIV Behavioral Surveillance system. Opioid-involved deaths are now roughly similar in magnitude to deaths during the peak of the HIV/AIDS epidemic, but these deaths have not elicited any comparable investment in data infrastructure.

The general lack of longitudinal data on people who use heroin and fentanyl creates problems for those trying to estimate the full cost of the crisis (e.g., understanding nonfatal overdoses), evaluate policy responses, and incorporate justifiable parameters into simulation models. The failure is also significant on the supply side. Although substantial resources go into research and monitoring with respect to health issues, much less effort is devoted to understanding the behavior of suppliers or measuring such fundamental parameters as prices and quantities.

There also are troubling delays in data reporting. Treatment admissions data can lag by more than two years and there also are noteworthy lags when it comes to releasing individual-level mortality data and seizure statistics. Such lags impede research and policy insights into this fast-moving problem (Ciccarone, 2017; Peiper et al., 2019).

Limiting Policy Responses to Existing Approaches Seems Unlikely to Reverse This Tide

In Chapter Two, we highlight how fentanyl and other synthetic opioids kill on a scale that is unprecedented among illegal drugs. The causes, dynamics, and likely future course are fundamentally different from other modern drug problems. These differences are not widely appreciated, and they matter in terms of how policymakers and society should respond. Existing strategies remain important, but they are not enough.

In this report, our goal is not to make specific policy recommendations or systematically assess costs and benefits, especially because the consequences of—and tradeoffs associated with—these policies would likely differ depending on the attributes of the jurisdiction in question. Rather, in Chapter Six, we advocate serious consideration of a broad array of innovative approaches to addressing the synthetic opioid crisis (e.g., supervised consumption sites; creative supply disruption; novel, evidence-informed treatment modalities).

The transition to fentanyl and other synthetic opioids is driven by suppliers, so it makes sense to consider supply reduction as one piece of a comprehensive effort. Even if supply cannot be eliminated altogether, delaying the entrenchment of fentanyl in a market by even a few years could save hundreds, if not thousands, of lives. Yet, there is a deserved rejection of some excesses of the recent past. There is little reason to believe that tougher sentences, including drug-induced homicide laws, for low-level retailers and easily replaceable functionaries (e.g., couriers) will make a positive difference (see, e.g., Kleiman, 2009). There is also little reason to believe that synthetic opioid production, which occurs mostly in China, could be curtailed in the short run (Pardo, Kilmer, and Huang, 2019).

But just as there are many types of harm reduction, there are many types of supply reduction—each with its own costs and benefits. Targeting importers and wholesalers of nearly pure fentanyl from China is very different from punishing street-level retailers who might not know the exact chemical or purity in what they sell. Additionally, not all efforts to impede supply would fill prisons. Internet sites play a prominent role in the trade of synthetic opioids; perhaps they could be shut down or spoofed. Other law enforcement efforts aimed at tracing the source of import through cyber investigations might be warranted in an era in which drugs can be transacted online without involving traditional organized criminal elements.

Innovation is necessitated by the nature and scale of the challenge brought by synthetic opioids, which, in their current forms and methods of marketing, represent a departure from previous crises. Indeed, it might be that this problem will eventually be resolved with approaches or technologies that do not currently exist or have yet to be tested. Limiting policy responses to existing approaches will likely be insufficient and may condemn many people to early deaths.

Acknowledgments

We are deeply indebted to the key informants who shared their experiences and insights with us during interviews. We also are very grateful for the detailed feedback we received from Lois Davis, Sara Duhachek Muggy, Vanda Felbab-Brown, Susan Gates, Sarah Mars, Leonard Pickard, Harold Pollack, and a reviewer who preferred to not be named. Rosalie Liccardo Pacula provided great insights during the early stages of this project. We would also like to thank Eugene Leventhal, who consulted with the research team as part of his independent work at Heinz College on the Estonian drug market. The views presented here are those of the authors alone.

Abbreviations

3MF	3-methylfentanyl
4-ANPP	4-anilino-N-phenethyl-4-piperidone
ADAM	Arrestee Drug Abuse Monitoring
BCCSU	British Columbia Center on Substance Use
CBP	U.S. Customs and Border Protection
CCENDU	Canadian Community Epidemiology Network on Drug Use
CDC	Centers for Disease Control and Prevention
CDT	dissuasion commission (Portugal)
DEA	U.S. Drug Enforcement Administration
DTO	drug trafficking organization
EMCDDA	European Monitoring Centre for Drugs and Drug Addiction
FSPP	Fentanyl Signature Profiling Program
FY	fiscal year
HAT	heroin-assisted treatment
HIV/AIDS	Human Immunodeficiency Virus/Acquired Immunodeficiency Syndrome
HSP	Heroin Signature Program
ICD	International Statistical Classification of Diseases and Related Health Problems
MCOD	multiple cause of death

MEC	medical examiners and coroners
MED	morphine-equivalent dose
NFLIS	National Forensic Laboratory Information System
NPP	N-phenethyl-4-piperidone
NSDUH	National Survey on Drugs and Health
ONDCP	Office of National Drug Control Policy
OUD	opioid use disorder
PWID	people who inject drugs
PWUD	people who use drugs
SAMHSA	Substance Abuse and Mental Health Services Administration
SSP	syringe service program
TOR	The Onion Router
UNODC	United Nations Office on Drugs and Crime
USPS	U.S. Postal Service
WHO	World Health Organization

CHAPTER ONE

Introduction

The number of opioid-involved fatalities in the United States is alarming. There were on the order of 50,000 opioid-involved overdose deaths in 2018, which is roughly similar in magnitude to the number of deaths from HIV/AIDS at its peak in 1995 (Centers for Disease Control and Prevention [CDC], 2013; Ruhm, 2018; Ahmad et al., 2019). The White House Council of Economic Advisers (2017) estimates that, in 2015 alone, the cost of the opioid epidemic exceeded $500 billion, largely because of lost productivity from premature death. These figures do not include secondary consequences, such as the psychological impacts on friends and family, especially on children, and the cost of injury from nonfatal overdose. Fewer experts have even considered the effects on first responder fatigue and the burden on emergency service provision.

This crisis is not the result of a single drug. Although the media and the public describe an opioid epidemic, it is more accurate to think of it as a series of overlapping and interrelated epidemics of pharmacologically similar substances—the opioid class of drugs. Ciccarone (2017, p. 107) refers to a "triple wave epidemic": The first wave was prescription opioids, the second wave was heroin, and the third—and ongoing—wave is synthetic opioids, such as fentanyl.

Fentanyl is not a new substance; it is used successfully in medicine. During the 1930s, German chemists synthesized meperidine—the first wholly synthetic analgesic comparable in strength to morphine (Eddy, 1957). The synthesis of methadone soon followed; the new chemical was used during the Second World War as a substitute for morphine

after Germany lost access to poppy (Booth, 1996). During the 1950s, the Belgian chemist Paul Janssen began studying meperidine to better understand its analgesic effects, leading to the synthesis of fentanyl in 1959 (López-Muñoz and Alamo, 2009).

Fentanyl was approved for use as an anesthetic in the United States in 1972. Its pharmacodynamics and ability to be made from inexpensive and readily available chemical precursors made it superior to morphine (Suzuki and El-Haddad, 2017). Fentanyl analogs, such as sufentanil, alfentanil, remifentanil, and carfentanil, were developed not long after fentanyl's synthesis (Armenian et al., 2018). Many of these synthetic opioids, including fentanyl, are highly potent full μ-opioid agonists that bind more efficiently to neuroreceptors than do other semisynthetic or natural opioids, such as codeine, morphine, oxycodone, or heroin (see Appendix A for more information). Active at doses of tens of micrograms for those without an opioid tolerance, they are some of the most potent substances developed (Suzuki and El-Haddad, 2017). Fentanyl's potency can range from 50 to 100 times that of morphine; several analogs, such as carfentanil, are reported to be 10,000 times more potent than morphine (Suzuki and El-Haddad, 2017). Other recently developed synthetic opioids have not yet been evaluated for their potency or pharmacokinetic properties (Armenian et al., 2018).[1] Their effects in humans are unknown. In addition, other pharmacological properties and physiological responses, such as fentanyl's ability to rapidly enter the brain and stiffen the muscles that control breathing (i.e., chest-wall rigidity), increase the risks of fatal overdose and respiratory depression (Gill et al., 2019).

The current wave of overdoses is largely attributable to illicitly manufactured fentanyl. Most of the fentanyl and novel synthetic opioids in U.S. street markets—as well as their precursor chemicals—originate in China, where the regulatory system does not effectively police the country's expansive pharmaceutical and chemical industries (Pardo, Kilmer, and Huang, 2019). According to federal law enforcement, synthetic opioids arrive in U.S. markets directly from Chinese manufacturers via the post, private couriers (e.g., UPS, FedEx), cargo,

---

[1]   This evolution is further discussed in Chapter Three.

by smugglers from Mexico, or by smugglers from Canada after being pressed into counterfeit prescription pills (O'Connor, 2017; Office of National Drug Control Policy [ONDCP], 2017). At this time, the share of synthetic opioids (such as fentanyl) that comes into the country through each point of entry is unknown. The U.S. Drug Enforcement Administration (DEA) suggests that some portion of fentanyl might be produced in Mexico using precursors from China (DEA, 2017b).

Synthetic opioids coming from China are much cheaper than Mexican heroin on a potency-adjusted basis (see, e.g., DEA, 2017b; Mars, Rosenblum, and Ciccarone, 2018; Rothberg and Stith, 2018). It is hard to tell precisely what the price differences are at the retail level because of drug mixing, variation in product types, and data constraints, but the gap from the dealers' perspective is clear. Recent RAND Corporation research identified multiple Chinese firms that are willing to ship 1 kg of nearly pure fentanyl to the United States for $2,000 to $5,000 (Pardo, Davis, and Moore, forthcoming). In terms of the morphine-equivalent dose (MED; a common method of comparing the strength of different opioids), a 95-percent pure kg of fentanyl at $5,000 would generally equate to less than $100 per MED kg.[2] For comparison, a 50-percent pure kg of Mexican heroin that costs $25,000 when exported to the United States would equate to at least $10,000 per MED kg. Thus, *heroin appears to be at least 100 times more expensive than fentanyl* in terms of MED at the import level.[3]

Objectives of This Report

Ten years ago, few would have predicted that illicitly manufactured fentanyl from abroad would sweep through British Columbia or parts of Appalachia and New England. As drug markets are flooded by fentanyl and other synthetic opioids, policymakers, researchers, and the public are trying to understand what to make of it and how to respond. Much as the synthesis of heroin in the late 19th century dis-

---

[2] For more information on MED and other terminology, see Appendix A.

[3] For more information on these calculations, see Appendix B.

placed morphine and forever changed the opiate landscape, the country might again be standing at the precipice of a new era: inexpensive, accessible, and mass-produced synthetic opioids could displace heroin. This might have important and hard-to-predict consequences for the broader drug policy landscape.

This mixed-methods report offers a systematic assessment of the past, present, and possible futures of fentanyl and other synthetic opioids found in illicit drug markets in the United States. Our goal, aimed at local, state, and national decisionmakers who are concerned about rising synthetic opioid overdose trends, is to provide insights and analyses that might improve their understanding of and responses to this problem. We also hope to provide new information to researchers, media sources, and other members of the public who are contributing to these critical policy discussions.

This analysis addresses the following questions:

- What can policymakers learn from U.S. fatal overdose and drug seizure trends?
- Why has fentanyl been so unevenly distributed across U.S. states and Canadian provinces?
- Why did fentanyl, which was first synthesized 60 years ago, create substantial problems only after 2013?
- What is the history of fentanyl outbreaks and why is today's outbreak much worse?
- What can be learned from other countries' experiences with synthetic opioids?
- What might the future of fentanyl and other synthetic opioids look like in the United States?
- What innovative policy options deserve discussion and analysis?
- How could surveillance and monitoring of synthetic opioids be improved?

Mixed-Methods Approach

This report uses multiple methods, incorporating a range of data collection and analysis activities. These methods are briefly described below; additional methodological details are offered in individual chapters.

Document Review

We reviewed the literature concerning the emergence of synthetic opioids in the United States and worldwide. These sources include, but are not limited to, the following areas:

- **literature on licit and illicit drug markets in the United States.** This literature includes sources commenting on the ongoing opioid epidemic, trends and topics pertaining to drug supply and demand in the United States, and associated responses.
- **literature on the drug situation in other jurisdictions.** This literature covers both academic sources and official documentation. Examples of the latter include, in the context of European Union countries, publications by the European Monitoring Centre for Drugs and Drug Addiction (EMCDDA), as well as information provided to the EMCDDA by national monitoring authorities.
- **literature on fentanyl and fentanyl outbreaks.** We conducted a review of documented fentanyl outbreaks in the United States, beginning in the late 1970s, to understand what factors were related to the introduction of these potent opioids in drug markets. We also summarized some of the published literature documenting the evolution of fentanyl synthesis over the past four decades.

Key Informant Interviews

We conducted 22 interviews with 25 individuals who are knowledgeable about synthetic opioids in selected international jurisdictions and/ or aspects of fentanyl markets in general (see Table 1.1). Informants include public officials working in the areas of drug policy or public health surveillance, practitioners working in the fields of public health and law enforcement, and researchers working on various aspects of

Table 1.1
Overview of Key Informants, by Stakeholder Group

Stakeholder Group	Number of Interviewees
Drug policy/surveillance officials	9
Law enforcement officials	9
Public health professionals	4
Researchers	3
Total	25

NOTE: Each interviewee was assigned to only one stakeholder group, which corresponds to the person's primary occupation. However, multiple interviewees could plausibly be categorized in different ways. For instance, numerous interviewed public health professionals also hold academic positions and engage in research.

drug policy. Interviews were semistructured, following a standardized interview template but allowing for the discussion of other topics. Interview notes were reviewed by members of the research team to identify emerging themes, which were then used to develop the structure for the discussion in Chapter Four. Further detail on these interviews is provided in Appendix E.

Secondary Data Analysis

We analyzed three data sets:

- **CDC mortality data.** We analyzed drug overdose mortality data between 2005 and 2017 from CDC. Per our agreement with CDC, we dropped jurisdiction-years with fewer than ten deaths. CDC's National Center for Health Statistics, in collaboration with the U.S. Census Bureau, reports annual population estimates by counties via the Bridged-Race Resident Population Estimates online tool (CDC, 2019). We used this tool to obtain annual county and state population estimates to calculate unadjusted or raw overdose death rates.
- **U.S. drug seizures data.** We examined publicly available drug seizure data at U.S. ports of entry, which are collected and reported by U.S. Customs and Border Protection (CBP); unclassified law enforcement reports from the DEA; and National Foren-

sic Laboratory Information System (NFLIS) reports for domestic drug seizures submitted by state and local forensic laboratories for 2007 and 2017. These data cover the entire country, allowing us to examine trends over time across states or counties.
- **international mortality and seizure data.** We reviewed data on drug-related deaths and drug seizures from the international jurisdictions discussed in this analysis. Where available, these data are presented alongside the discussion of the respective national drug market.

Structure of This Report

In Chapter Two, we offer a detailed analysis of individual-level overdose mortality data and state-specific drug seizure information in the United States. Given the sudden rise of fentanyl and other synthetic opioids, in Chapter Three, we offer insights about why a drug first synthesized 60 years ago is only now creating a crisis in North America. In Chapter Four, we look beyond the United States to assess how synthetic opioid problems have (or have not) developed in five other countries: Canada, Estonia, Finland, Latvia, and Sweden. We provide a detailed summary of the market characteristics and variations across countries and of factors associated with the emergence of synthetic opioids, as well as lessons for the United States. In Chapter Five, we draw on the results of our analyses and the literature summaries presented in Chapter Four to posit a series of possible scenarios for the future of synthetic opioids in the United States. In Chapter Six, we synthesize insights from these analyses and offer ideas intended to inform policy discussions and future research.

CHAPTER TWO

Insights From Mortality and Seizure Data in the United States

As discussed in the introduction, overdoses in North America continue to rise as potent synthetic opioids, such as fentanyl, make their way into drug markets. To better understand the shifting landscape brought on by the arrival of synthetic opioids, this chapter examines U.S. trends in both mortality data and supply-side indicators from law enforcement.

Both types of data have significant limitations, so patterns observed in just one type of data might be suspect. However, the two data sources' limitations are largely unrelated, so when the two signal similar trends in the same places and times, they are more likely to reflect true underlying market trends. In this chapter, we do indeed find considerable overlap in temporal and spatial trends for synthetic opioid overdoses and supply-side measures.

In brief, both data sources show rapid increases in indicators; a sharp east-west divide, with the most affected areas all being in the eastern United States; and great variation even within the eastern United States. The overdose data alone suggest that, in some markets, synthetic opioids might have begun to replace heroin, rather than only adulterate it.[1] The law enforcement data alone show growth in the range of substances, from just fentanyl to multiple types of synthetic opioids, albeit with fentanyl still dominant. For more information on

---

[1] In this case, some heroin dealers have mixed fentanyl into the retail heroin supply in order to increase the desired opioid-like effects while reducing the amount of heroin needed.

synthetic opioids and their terminology and conversions to adjust for potency, see Appendix A.

Drug Overdose Fatalities

Data Sources and Limitations

CDC collects death certificates from state and local medical examiners' and coroners' (MECs') offices and consolidates those documents to create its multiple cause of death (MCOD) data series. Using the MCOD data, we were able to examine individual overdose deaths. The capacity of MECs to accurately determine drug overdose deaths varies. A recent survey of MECs across the United States notes variation in the frequency of toxicological examinations and available resources (DEA NFLIS, 2018). According to the survey, in 2016, less than 60 percent of MECs always conduct a toxicology examination for fentanyl or fentanyl-related substances. Scholl and colleagues (2018) notes that data from 27 states meet very good to excellent drug overdose death reporting criteria. Other research has noted the variation in drug overdose death counts, with some states reporting increasing shares of unknown or unspecified drugs in overdoses, rendering trend analyses difficult (Ruhm, 2018). It is highly likely that some states are undercounting the magnitude of the synthetic opioid overdose problem.

Another limitation is that multiple drugs might be reported in the decedent's death certificate as *underlying* causes of death. We analyzed individual death record information, allowing us to examine the share of drug overdoses containing multiple underlying drug poisonings. However, in these cases, it is impossible to point to any single cause of death or determine whether drugs were consumed at the same time. For example, someone who regularly uses prescription opioids could turn to the heroin market to avoid withdrawal after failing to obtain prescription medications for a couple of days. In this example, the heroin consumed would be adulterated with fentanyl, causing the individual to succumb to a fatal overdose. Upon toxicological analysis, the medical examiner might report three separate underlying drug poisoning causes of death: semisynthetic/natural opioids, heroin, and synthetic opioids. Without knowing more information than what is shown in the toxicological analysis, we cannot determine the sequencing of drugs used, only that all were present.

National overdose death data, which use the 10th revision of the International Statistical Classification of Diseases and Related Health Problems (ICD-10), lump all synthetic opioids other than methadone into one poisoning code (T40.4), making it impossible for those who lack access to original death records to determine the specific chemical that contributed to a fatality. That said, a 2018 textual analysis of death records by CDC shows that most synthetic opioid overdoses through 2016 involved fentanyl (Hedegaard, Miniño, and Warner, 2018). See Appendix D for greater detail on data and methods for analyzing drug overdose deaths and seizures.

To complicate this issue further, fentanyl itself is a prescription medication. Overdose death records do not allow us to determine the source of the drug involved in death. However, as mentioned earlier, we can infer that most of the deaths involving fentanyl are from illicit sources because prescription levels have not increased, while seizures of illicitly manufactured product have (Gladden, Martinez, and Seth, 2016).

National Trends

Between 2013 and 2017, the rate of overdose death records mentioning synthetic opioids increased from one per 100,000 people to nine per 100,000, which is approximately double the corresponding 2017 rates for heroin (4.9 per 100,000 people) or prescription opioids (4.4 per 100,000 people; Hedegaard, Miniño, and Warner, 2018). Although the prescription opioid rate was higher than other categories between 2007 and 2014, the rate of overdose deaths involving heroin or synthetic opioids surpassed those involving prescription opioids by 2015 (see Figure 2.1).

However, Figure 2.1 obscures the diffusion of synthetic opioids across other drug classes because one death can involve multiple drugs. Because synthetic opioids often appear as adulterants in other drugs—specifically, heroin—Figure 2.1 shows the U.S. drug overdose death

Figure 2.1
U.S. Drug Overdose Death Rates per 100,000 People, by Year and Drug Category

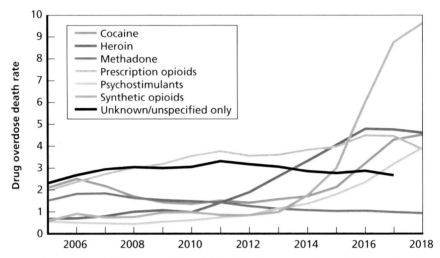

SOURCE: Data for this figure are from deidentified MCOD certificate files produced by the National Center for Health Statistics, 2005–2017, shared with RAND researchers under a data use agreement.
NOTE: The rates for 2018 are provisional and subject to change.

counts between 2005 and 2017 for various drugs, separating out those for which a synthetic opioid was present in death certificate records.

Figure 2.2 shows the number of overdose deaths involving synthetic opioids (to avoid double counting, we have excluded deaths that also mention cocaine, heroin, prescription opioids, or psychostimulants from the "synthetic opioid only" panel). Beginning in 2014, the number of overdose deaths—across all drug death categories—involving synthetic opioids began to climb, with steep increases in 2016 and 2017.

By 2017, more than half of the 15,000 heroin overdose deaths in the United States involved synthetic opioids. What is perhaps more surprising is that the same is true for cocaine; by 2017, a little more than half of fatal cocaine overdose death records also mentioned synthetic opioids. The share of overdose records involving psychostimulants (generally methamphetamine) that also mentioned synthetic opi-

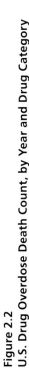
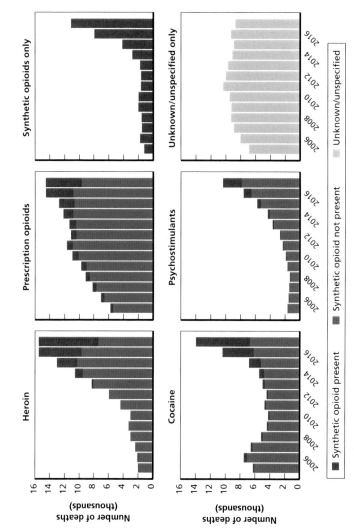

Figure 2.2
U.S. Drug Overdose Death Count, by Year and Drug Category

SOURCE: Data for this figure are from deidentified public-use MCOD certificate files produced by the National Center for Health Statistics, 2005–2017, shared with RAND researchers under a data use agreement.
NOTE: The "synthetic opioids only" panel excludes deaths that also mention cocaine, heroin, prescription opioids, or psychostimulants.

oids grew more slowly, but by 2017, one in four psychostimulant deaths involved synthetic opioids.

Counts of unknown or unspecified overdoses have declined from their peak in 2011 as states have improved drug overdose reporting. Nevertheless, several states continue to report large shares of unspecified drug overdose deaths.[2] However, without knowing how frequently medical authorities test for fentanyl metabolites over time, we are unable to determine what share of the increases in synthetic opioid overdoses is due to more-robust toxicological exams versus increased supply.

The share of psychostimulant overdoses involving synthetic opioids might be much higher than the share of psychostimulant use episodes involving synthetic opioids. Stimulant users might not be opioid-tolerant, and the rate of overdose per use session thus could be higher than when stimulants, such as cocaine and methamphetamine, are consumed alone.

Data from Ohio provide a small window into this possibility. As we discuss later, 70 percent of cocaine overdose cases in Ohio in 2017 also mentioned synthetic opioids (compared with the national average of about 50 percent), but only 12 percent of retail-level cocaine samples obtained by law enforcement were found to include fentanyl (Cauchon, 2019). Interestingly, none of the larger cocaine samples contained fentanyl, implying that fentanyl entered the cocaine supply at lower market levels within the state, rather than from further up the distribution chain. The 70-percent and 12-percent figures are not directly comparable. The former percentage pertains to what was detected in the bodies of decedents, some of whom might have consumed two separate packages of drugs, one with cocaine only and one that contained fentanyl. Furthermore, the overdose data pertain to all synthetic opi-

---

[2] Pennsylvania is perhaps a constructive example. That state, which has witnessed a doubling in overdose deaths since 2014, has reported unknown or unspecified overdose deaths in numbers that are two or three times those for heroin. The rate of these uncategorized overdose deaths in Pennsylvania, which remained stable between 2005 and 2013, has doubled since 2014, when fentanyl started to enter illicit drug markets. As of 2017, these deaths outnumber heroin-involved and synthetic opioid–involved overdoses by factors of three and 1.25, respectively. This suggests substantial measurement error in overdose death reporting.

oids other than methadone, whereas the laboratory analysis of cocaine samples was described as testing specifically for fentanyl. Still, the gap is stark.

As explained in Cauchon (2019), there are two theories for how fentanyl gets into cocaine. One is that dealers intentionally add the fentanyl to cocaine, creating what amounts to a prepackaged speedball. The other, which Cauchon terms the "sloppy dealer theory," involves accidental contamination by dealers who sell both cocaine and heroin. In this case, the heroin is intentionally adulterated with fentanyl, while the cocaine is contaminated accidentally. Without knowing the purity of fentanyl or analogs present in seizures, it is hard to say whether samples that test positive for synthetic opioids involve only residue left over from cutting other drugs or intentional mixing by drug retailers.[3]

Variation Across States in Synthetic Opioid Overdose Fatalities

Patterns of synthetic opioid overdose are far from uniform across the country. As mentioned earlier, CDC rated 35 states as maintaining good (8) or very good to excellent (27) overdose death reporting in 2017.[4] We concentrate on results for those 35 states.

We consider two types of outcomes in each case, contrasting values for 2014 and 2017 (the latest year for which individual-level data were available). The first outcome is the rate of overdose deaths mentioning synthetic opioids per 100,000 people (see Figure 2.3). This is perhaps the most direct measure of the severity of the synthetic opioid problem. The second outcome, shown in Figures 2.4 and 2.5, is the proportion of heroin and cocaine overdose deaths, respectively, that also mention synthetic opioids.

---

[3] A person who sells drugs might not clean surfaces or equipment properly when diluting street drugs, leading to cross-contamination and unintentional mixing. For example, after adulterating heroin with fentanyl on his kitchen table, a drug dealer might haphazardly wipe down the surface before diluting cocaine with caffeine. Such sloppiness could result in unintentional cocaine and fentanyl mixtures because minute quantities of fentanyl residue might remain on the surface.

[4] States with good reporting had 80 to 90 percent of drug overdose death records mention at least one specific drug in 2016; for states with very good to excellent reporting, the corresponding rate was more than or equal to 90 percent (Scholl et al., 2018).

Figure 2.3
Synthetic Opioid Overdose Death Rate per 100,000 People in the United States, 2014 and 2017

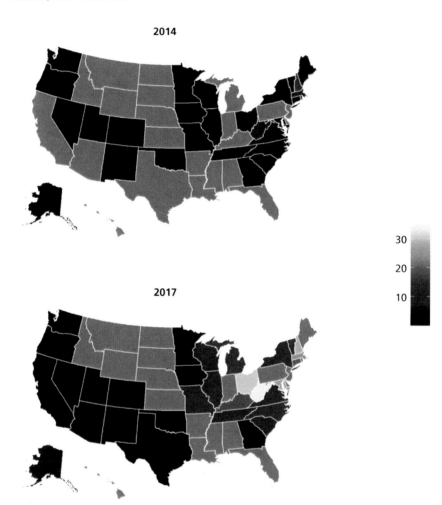

SOURCE: Data for this figure are from deidentified MCOD certificate files produced by the National Center for Health Statistics, 2005–2017, shared with RAND researchers under a data use agreement.
NOTE: States in gray have only fair overdose reporting.

Figure 2.4
Heroin Overdose Deaths Involving Synthetic Opioids, by State, 2014 and 2017

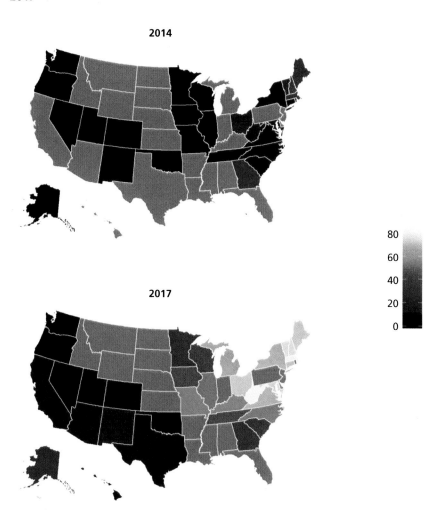

SOURCE: Data for this figure are from deidentified MCOD certificate files produced by the National Center for Health Statistics, 2005–2017, shared with RAND researchers under a data use agreement.
NOTE: States in gray have only fair overdose reporting.

Figure 2.5
Cocaine Overdose Deaths Involving Synthetic Opioids, by State, 2014 and 2017

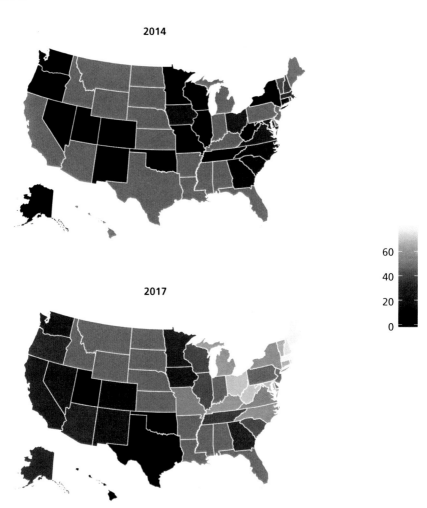

SOURCE: Data for this figure are from deidentified MCOD certificate files produced by the National Center for Health Statistics, 2005–2017, shared with RAND researchers under a data use agreement.
NOTE: States in gray have only fair overdose reporting.

All three figures suggest that exposure to synthetic opioids is much more common in the eastern half of the country and that the east-west gap grew from 2014 to 2017. The western half of the United States did not see a rapid explosion in synthetic opioid overdose deaths from 2014 to 2017, while the same cannot be said for states in the eastern half of the country. That is, synthetic opioids appeared first in the east, and the next three years saw further acceleration of the issue in that region rather than the west "catching up."

Likewise, all three figures show that synthetic opioid seizures and deaths are most concentrated in parts of Appalachia, New England, and the Midatlantic. In Figure 2.3, the ten states with the highest synthetic opioid overdose death rates in 2017 are, in order: West Virginia, Ohio, New Hampshire, Maryland, Massachusetts, Maine, Connecticut, Rhode Island, Delaware, and Kentucky. According to Scholl et al. (2018), all of these states except Delaware and Kentucky have very good to excellent overdose death reporting. Although these ten states constituted 12 percent of the country's population, they made up 35 percent of the 28,500 fatal overdoses involving synthetic opioids in 2017. Ohio's share of fatalities alone was almost 12.5 percent, while the state made up about 3.5 percent of the country's total population.

Figure 2.4 shows a substantial increase in the proportion of heroin overdose deaths that also involve synthetic opioids. By 2017, it was rare in Massachusetts or West Virginia for heroin overdose deaths to not involve synthetic opioids. The pattern for cocaine in Figure 2.5 is similar but is slightly delayed and less pronounced.

Suggestions That Synthetic Opioids Might Be Displacing Heroin
We examined the trends shown in Figures 2.4 and 2.5 in greater detail by replicating Figure 2.2 at the state level for three states that are acutely affected and that have very good to excellent overdose death reporting: West Virginia, Ohio, and New Hampshire.[5] These states were among the first to be exposed to synthetic opioids, have the highest overdose death rates, and experienced the fentanyl phenomenon somewhat dif-

---

[5] Per our data use agreement with CDC, we removed state-year death rates with fewer than ten deaths from these plots.

ferently. In particular, New Hampshire's mortality data suggest that synthetic opioids have largely supplanted other drug-involved overdose deaths, and the other two states show varying degrees of overdose combinations.

Figure 2.6 shows the overdose death rates for West Virginia, which had the highest synthetic opioid overdose rate in 2017 and also had high rates of non-medical use of prescription opioids and overdose. Some instances of prescription opioids co-occurring with synthetic opioids could pertain to prescribed synthetic opioids (e.g., transdermal fentanyl patches or tramadol), particularly in the early years. Synthetic opioids began showing up in illicit drugs around 2014. By 2017, in West Virginia, about 80 percent of heroin overdose deaths, 70 percent of cocaine overdose deaths, and 45 percent of prescription opioid overdose deaths (which have been declining in the state since 2014) involved synthetic opioids.

Ohio had the second-highest synthetic opioid overdose death rate in the country in 2017. Figure 2.7 shows similarities with West Virginia but also shows differences, including a substantially lower rate of deaths involving prescription opioids and a downturn in heroin overdose deaths in 2017. West Virginia—and, indeed, the country as a whole—showed declines in heroin overdose deaths that did not also mention synthetic opioids, but in Ohio, the total number of deaths mentioning heroin actually fell in 2017 for the first time since 2009, and, at the time of this writing, there are few heroin overdose deaths in Ohio that exclude synthetic opioids. This suggests that, in heroin markets in Ohio, synthetic opioids could be replacing—rather than augmenting—heroin. Other sources have reported a similar trend (e.g., Daniulaityte et al., 2017). Indeed, the reach of synthetic opioids is not just affecting those who only use heroin. In 2017, about 70 percent of cocaine and psychostimulant overdoses and about half of prescription opioid overdoses in Ohio also mentioned synthetic opioids.

New Hampshire had the third-highest overdose death rate in 2017 involving synthetic opioids. What stands out is its synthetic opioid–only deaths, which are even more prevalent than in Ohio (a little more than 20 per 100,000 people in New Hampshire compared with about 12 per 100,000 in Ohio). In New Hampshire, heroin and prescription

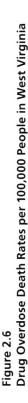

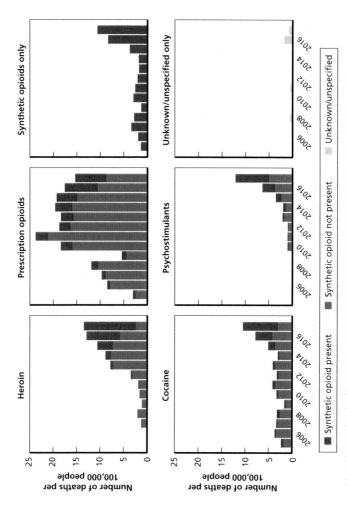

Figure 2.6
Drug Overdose Death Rates per 100,000 People in West Virginia

SOURCE: Data for this figure are from deidentified MCOD certificate files produced by the National Center for Health Statistics, 2005–2017, shared with RAND researchers under a data use agreement.
NOTE: The "synthetic opioids only" panel excludes deaths that also mention cocaine, heroin, prescription opioids, or psychostimulants.

Figure 2.7
Drug Overdose Death Rates per 100,000 People in Ohio

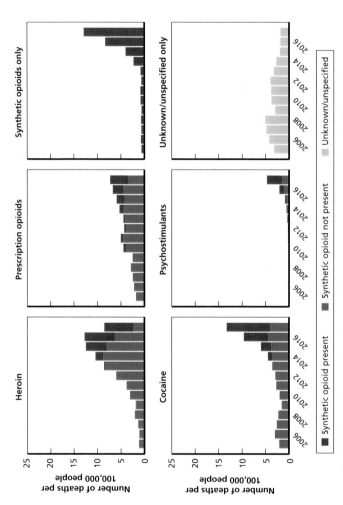

SOURCE: Data for this figure are from deidentified MCOD certificate files produced by the National Center for Health Statistics, 2005–2017, shared with RAND researchers under a data use agreement.
NOTE: The "synthetic opioids only" panel excludes deaths that also mention cocaine, heroin, prescription opioids, or psychostimulants.

opioid overdoses have been declining since their peaks in 2014, albeit at lower levels than in West Virginia or Ohio. In 2017, three-quarters of overdose deaths in New Hampshire from heroin, cocaine, or psychostimulants and about one-third of those from prescription opioids also involved synthetic opioids. Because only one-quarter of heroin overdoses do not mention synthetic opioids and total heroin overdoses have fallen so far, there are now very few heroin-only overdoses in New Hampshire, suggesting that heroin without synthetic opioids is now somewhat uncommon there (see Figure 2.8).

In sum, this analysis of overdose mortality data through 2017 shows that several regional markets are increasingly transitioning toward synthetic opioids and away from traditional illicit opioids, such as heroin and diverted prescription pain relievers. Additionally, an increasing share of cocaine overdoses also involves synthetic opioids.

Full data are only available through 2017, but national provisional data for 2018 indicate a continued increase in deaths involving synthetic opioids (Ahmad et al., 2019).

Supply-Side Indicators

Data Sources and Limitations

In this section, we describe trends using a variety of unclassified and public law enforcement or "supply side" data series from CBP, the DEA's NFLIS, and the DEA's own seizure data. These supply indicators generally show how drug markets are changing in terms of what substances might be offered and where. Such indicators often are used to help law enforcement inform interdiction responses.

Data on drug seizures have limitations. They are not representative samples of the supply of drugs and might be influenced by changes in law enforcement policies. When problems with a new drug increase, one might expect that drug to get greater attention from law enforcement, so seizures might increase more quickly than does the actual level of supply or use. That dynamic has always been a challenge, even with traditional drugs, such as cocaine or heroin (Reuter, 1995). Synthetic opioids add another wrinkle because the number of forensic

Figure 2.8
Drug Overdose Death Rates per 100,000 People in New Hampshire

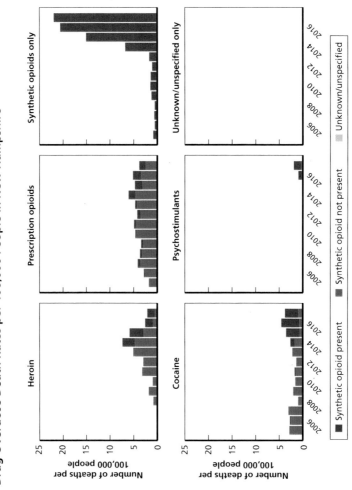

SOURCE: Data for this figure are from deidentified MCOD certificate files produced by the National Center for Health Statistics, 2005–2017, shared with RAND researchers under a data use agreement.
NOTE: The "synthetic opioids only" panel excludes deaths that also mention cocaine, heroin, prescription opioids, or psychostimulants.

laboratories that routinely test for these relatively new substances has grown over time. Thus, the number of synthetic opioid seizures might have grown faster than the underlying supply, and the proportion of those seizures that is tested and identified as containing synthetic opioids might also have grown.

In general, these three public data sources offer mere counts of the number of samples containing a particular chemical, not the underlying data. This limits our ability to adjust for weight, purity, or drugs appearing in combination. For example, two separate seizures, one of heroin and one of fentanyl, could contribute the same number to these counts as one seizure that contained heroin adulterated with fentanyl. These data cannot distinguish between instances in which a bag of heroin has a trace of fentanyl and a bag of fentanyl contains a trace of heroin, nor can they determine whether a drug was added intentionally or is present only because of residual contamination (e.g., sloppy drug mixing or accidental contamination from reusing surfaces and paraphernalia).

These limitations are not insignificant, but, as mentioned in the introduction, they are different from and mostly unrelated to the limitations in the overdose data. Thus, seizure data provide a complementary view to what is seen in overdose data, and where the two sources agree, one might suspect that they reflect some true underlying trends.

Customs and Border Protection Seizure Trends
CBP serves as the main law enforcement arm in detecting and interdicting drugs and other contraband that enter the United States through air or land ports of entry or across the southwest border. Other available law enforcement data provide counts, but CBP data describe weights seized. These are *bulk weights*, meaning the total weight of a mixture containing fentanyl, not adjusted for purity. So two 1-kg seizures—one that is 5 percent fentanyl by weight and one that is 95 percent fentanyl—show up the same way in these data.

The CBP seizure data show a rising trend in the bulk weight of seizures containing fentanyl for fiscal years (FYs) 2015 to 2019 (see Table 2.1). Seizures were quite modest in FY 2015, with just 32 kg seized by CBP, but they increased tenfold by FY 2016, almost tripled in

Table 2.1
CBP Seizures of Fentanyl, FYs 2015–2019

CBP Office	FY 2015	FY 2016	FY 2017	FY 2018	FY 2019[a]
Field Operations	32	271	852	811	322
Border Patrol	0	48	82	176	52
Total	32	319	935	988	374

SOURCE: CBP, 2019a.
NOTES: All numbers are in kilograms. Numbers are not adjusted for purity.
[a] FY 2019 data are through February 2019.

FY 2017, and then increased slightly in FY 2018. The rise in reported seizures lagged behind the increase in overdose deaths described earlier; overdose deaths were already increasing in FY 2014–2015.

The totals in Table 2.1 are not adjusted for purity, which is often low for seizures of drugs arriving at land border crossings and very high for seizures of drugs arriving by mail or express consignment operator (e.g., FedEx, DHL) (DEA NFLIS, 2018). Indeed, CBP notes that, "in many cases, trace amounts of fentanyl are part of mixed loads passing through the [southwest border]" (CBP, 2019b, p. 7).

In Table 2.2, we break down CBP's FY 2018 seizures of fentanyl by mode of transport and estimate their purity-adjusted weight based on purity measures provided by the DEA. In particular, we multiply bulk weights by 90 percent if the drugs seized arrived by air, mail, or express consignment. We multiplied by 7.5 percent for seizures that arrived by land or were reported by the U.S. Border Patrol. The latter two modes of transport account for 83 percent of the bulk weight but just 30 percent of the fentanyl, after making this adjustment for purity. It is not entirely clear why seizures of shipments arriving by land are of such low purity. Pardo, Davis, and Moore (forthcoming) mentions several possibilities, such as drug trafficking organizations (DTOs) mixing fentanyl with diluents prior to smuggling (either in powder or pressed into counterfeit tablets) or synthesizing product of low purity.

As shown in Table 2.2, the majority of seizures occur at mail facilities, with the average weight amounting to less than 150 g. Seizures of fentanyl at express consignment facilities are heavier than those that arrive by mail, at almost 700 g on average. Land seizures are the bulki-

Table 2.2
CBP Seizures of Fentanyl in FY 2018, by Mode of Transport

Mode of Transport	Weight (kg)	Estimated Purity-Adjusted Weight (kg)	Number of Seizure Events	Average Weight of Seizure (bulk kg)
Land (mostly southwest border)	654.00	49.05	182	3.59
Border patrol	176.36	13.23	—	—
Express consignment	52.62	47.36	76	0.69
Mail	61.72	55.55	455	0.14
Air (other)	50.06	45.05	2	25.03
Total	994.76	210.24	715	—

SOURCE: CBP, 2019a.
NOTE: The purity of fentanyl arriving at mail and express consignment facilities is often 90 percent, while seizures at the southwest border are reportedly 5- to 10-percent pure; here we use the midpoint of 7.5-percent pure. CBP did not report the number of Border Patrol seizure events, so we cannot calculate the average weight.

est, weighing more than 3.5 kg. These variations, as well as the noted purity disparity between seizures arriving by land and air, suggest variation across supply modes.

National Forensic Laboratory Trends Across Region and Time

DEA NFLIS collects data from forensic labs analyzing drug samples for state and local law enforcement agencies. The data span 2007 to 2017 and come from the entire United States. Some laboratories do not participate, but coverage is high, increasing from about 88 percent of all drug crime labs participating in 2007 to 98 percent in 2017 (DEA NFLIS, 2019). Most samples are from seizures, but material is also obtained through undercover purchases and miscellaneous methods.

In this section, we describe trends in the state-year counts of samples containing particular chemicals. Without analyzing individual seizure events, we are unable to adjust for purity or evaluate drug mixtures (e.g., heroin containing fentanyl), location, or where in the supply chain the seizure occurred (e.g., wholesale versus retail).

In brief, the NFLIS counts show extraordinarily rapid growth over time; domination by fentanyl itself as opposed to other synthetic opioids, such as furanyl fentanyl; fentanyl's growth preceding the growth of less common synthetic opioids by a year or two; and sharp geographic concentration, mostly in the same states that recorded the most overdose deaths associated with synthetic opioids.

These trends mirror those described earlier for overdose deaths, albeit with a slight delay, but it is impossible to know whether they reflect changes in market trends as opposed to changes in law enforcement priorities and laboratory protocols. It seems plausible that, precisely in those times and places where synthetic opioid problems truly were growing, law enforcement might have worked harder to seize substances and forensic labs might have been more likely to test for them. If so, the trends in NFLIS might be exaggerated relative to true underlying market trends.

Although it is impossible to rule out the possibility that some trends in NFLIS data are merely artifacts of changing enforcement or testing practices, we believe that the trends are suggestive and value their specificity in terms of particular chemicals. Whereas the MCOD overdose death data lump together all synthetic opioids other than methadone, NFLIS data distinguish among scores of different specific chemicals.

In particular, between 2007 and 2017, NFLIS recorded more than 150,000 counts of fentanyl and fentanyl-related substances. Table 2.3 shows that the vast majority of reported substances were specifically fentanyl (79.5 percent), with furanyl fentanyl (5.2 percent), and carfentanil (4.8 percent) showing up as the second- and third-most-common chemicals. The other category includes 37 fentanyl-related chemicals that were reported in NFLIS but in counts fewer than 1,000.

Figure 2.9 demonstrates the extraordinary rise in the number of law enforcement samples that NFLIS records as containing fentanyl or a fentanyl-related substance between 2007 and 2017. For fentanyl itself, counts went from 978 in 2013 to more than 59,000 in 2017 (DEA, 2018e). There was also a noticeable jump in counts of other fentanyl-related substances, such as furanyl fentanyl and carfentanil, but somewhat later; they were not reported in NFLIS prior to 2016. A similar and contemporaneous phenomenon of increasing seizures of

Table 2.3
Fentanyl and Fentanyl-Related Substances Reported to NFLIS, 2007–2017

Chemical	Count
Fentanyl	119,607
Furanyl fentanyl	7,763
Carfentanil	7,155
Acetyl fentanyl	5,562
Acryl fentanyl	2,084
4-Fluoroisobutyryl fentanyl	1,646
Cyclopropyl fentanyl	1,445
3-Methylfentanyl	1,190
Other	3,929
Total	150,381

SOURCE: DEA NFLIS reports, 2007–2017.

Figure 2.9
Drug Seizures of Fentanyl and Fentanyl-Related Substances in the United States, 2007–2017

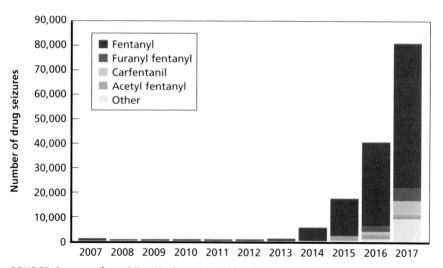

SOURCE: Data are from DEA NFLIS reports, 2007–2017.

fentanyl-related substances has been reported in Canada and parts of Europe (see Chapter Four).

Figure 2.10 plots the number of counts for less common fentanyl-related substances (i.e., chemicals other than fentanyl, furanyl fentanyl, carfentanil, or acetyl fentanyl). NFLIS reported no counts of these chemicals prior to 2014 and just a handful of instances of butyryl fentanyl in 2014. Counts remained relatively low and then exploded from fewer than 900 in 2016 to more than 9,000 in 2017. Between 2014 and 2017, the most-frequently reported fentanyl analogs besides furanyl fentanyl, carfentanil, and acetyl fentanyl were acryl fentanyl (2,084), 4-fluoroisobutyryl fentanyl (1,646), cyclopropyl fentanyl (1,445), and 3-methylfentanyl (1,190). None of these substances have recognized medical utility, and some, such as 3-methylfentanyl, are more potent than fentanyl and have been subject to control for quite some time. Others are entirely new and might not be listed in drug control laws. As we discuss later, chemical variation could generate additional harms

Figure 2.10
Drug Seizures of Less Common Fentanyl-Related Substances in the United States, 2014–2017

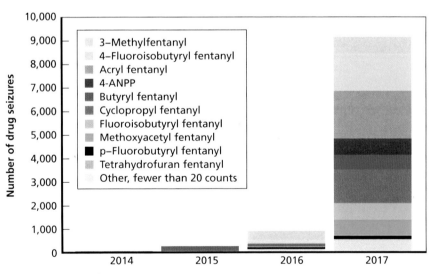

SOURCE: Data are from DEA NFLIS reports, 2007–2017.
NOTE: 4-ANPP = 4-anilino-N-phenethyl-4-piperidone.

in that dealers and users might not know the effects of these substances, let alone how to dose them in appropriate quantities. Furthermore, the constant churning of available chemicals impedes users' and sellers' ability to adapt to increased harms.

There is considerable geographic variation in seizures containing fentanyl and fentanyl-related substances, with parts of New England and Appalachia reporting the highest numbers to NFLIS. Table 2.4 shows the top ten states for counts of fentanyl and fentanyl-related substances reported to NFLIS. They largely mirror the states with the highest drug overdose death rates involving synthetic opioids, with one exception. West Virginia—the state with the highest synthetic opioid overdose death rate in 2017—is conspicuously absent from Table 2.4.

Figure 2.11 shows that, for states spanning Appalachia, the Midatlantic, and New England, there is generally a positive correlation between states' rates of synthetic opioid seizures and their per capita counts of fentanyl and fentanyl-related substances submitted to NFLIS in 2017. The one conspicuous outlier is West Virginia. Scholl et al. (2018) rates two states' overdose data as fair (Pennsylvania and New

Table 2.4
Top Ten States for Counts of Fentanyl and Fentanyl-Related Substances Reported to NFLIS, 2007–2017

State	Count
Ohio	41,118
Massachusetts	17,631
Pennsylvania	15,899
New Jersey	10,854
Maryland	6,634
New York	6,343
Virginia	6,216
Illinois	5,479
Florida	5,124
New Hampshire	5,083
Total	120,381

SOURCE: DEA NFLIS reports, 2007–2017.

Figure 2.11
Synthetic Opioid Overdose Death Rates Plotted Versus 2017 per Capita NFLIS Fentanyl and Fentanyl-Related Counts for Parts of Appalachia, the Midatlantic, and New England

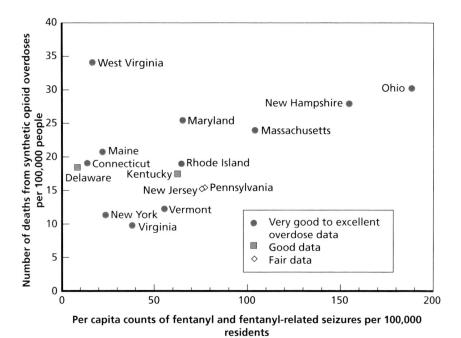

SOURCES: Seizure data are from DEA NFLIS reports, 2007–2017; overdose data are from deidentified MCOD certificate files produced by the National Center for Health Statistics and shared with RAND researchers under a data use agreement.

Jersey). These two states are below the trend line, but not dramatically so.

Figure 2.12 shows the per capita rate of fentanyl and fentanyl-related counts by state over time for the entire United States. It confirms the earlier finding from the overdose data that the synthetic opioid problem is concentrated in the eastern half of the country.

One of the great strengths of the NFLIS data is their ability to distinguish among the many different types of synthetic opioids, whereas the CDC MCOD data lump them together. As shown in Figure 2.13, in some states (e.g., Massachusetts and New Hampshire), fentanyl appears to dominate the counts reported to NFLIS, whereas

Figure 2.12
Fentanyl and Fentanyl-Related Seizure Counts per 100,000 Residents,
2014–2017

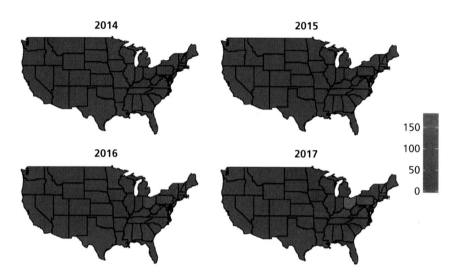

SOURCE: Data are from DEA NFLIS reports, 2007–2017.

other states (e.g., New Jersey and Ohio) detect a wider variety of synthetic opioids, with fentanyl analogs making up more than 40 percent of counts reported to NFLIS in recent years. Indeed, finer distinctions can be drawn. In 2017, New Jersey reported many furanyl fentanyl exhibits, but in Ohio, the super-potent opioid carfentanil was more common.

Variation in types of synthetic opioids might exacerbate the already high risks that people who use drugs face. Even if users are aware that their drugs are adulterated with some type of synthetic opioid, they (as well as the dealer) might not be aware of the morphine milligram equivalency of that particular analog (Mars, Rosenblum, and Ciccarone, 2018). Ohio's staggering overdose counts may be in part because of the rising share of carfentanil showing up in seizures. This is similar to considerations reported in other countries facing variability in their fentanyl markets, as is discussed in Chapter Four.

Figure 2.13
Fentanyl and Fentanyl-Related Seizure Counts in Selected States

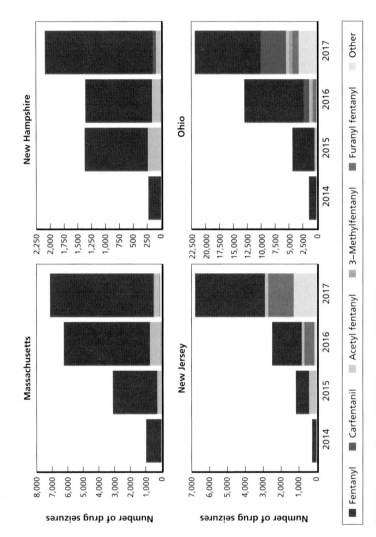

SOURCE: Data are from DEA NFLIS reports, 2007–2017.
NOTE: Scales on y-axis are different across states.

One of the intriguing findings from the overdose data is the possibility that, in some places (e.g., New Hampshire), fentanyl might be driving heroin out of the market, rather than just being added to it. To pursue that idea further, in Figure 2.14, we compare per capita seizure counts for heroin and all fentanyl and fentanyl-related substances (labeled as "fentanyls" in the figure) in Massachusetts, New Hampshire, Ohio, and West Virginia. Because these are NFLIS state-year counts, we are unable to determine the overlap in seizures that contain both heroin and fentanyl.[6] However, analysis of NFLIS data by the DEA suggests that, between 2014 and 2016, about 70 percent of exhibits containing fentanyl or fentanyl-related substances contained only fentanyl or analogs; only about one-quarter contained heroin (DEA NFLIS, 2018). Nonetheless, in all four states, per capita heroin seizure counts began to decline around 2014, while counts for fentanyls increased each year, starting in 2013 or 2014. Fentanyls overtook heroin counts in all states except for West Virginia, starting with New Hampshire in 2015.

This is additional circumstantial evidence that, in these acutely affected markets, fentanyls might be displacing heroin. It is important corroborating evidence precisely because synthetic opioids can be so much deadlier than heroin. If synthetic opioids dominate overdose cases, that conflates how often they are used with the rate of overdose per session of use. Seizure data might suffer a parallel bias if police try harder to seize synthetic opioids than they do to seize heroin, but that seems unlikely. Some states suffering from exposure to fentanyl are still in transition. Seizure counts of heroin or fentanyl are showing up in equal amounts in Kentucky, and roughly half of the overdose deaths in that state also mention synthetic opioids.

DEA Seizures That Could Reflect Activities at Higher Market Levels

NFLIS counts are not adjusted for the weight or size of samples, so they are dominated by smaller, retail activities. The DEA also seizes and analyzes fentanyl exhibits and customarily focuses on higher levels

---

[6] In the NFLIS data, a single drug seizure containing both heroin and fentanyl would be counted twice, once for heroin and once for fentanyl.

Figure 2.14
Per Capita Counts of Heroin and Fentanyl Reported to NFLIS, 2012–2017

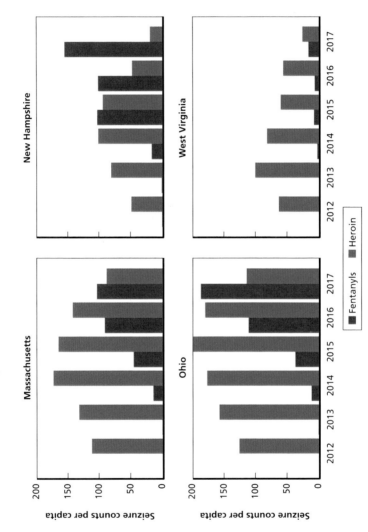

SOURCE: Data are from DEA NFLIS reports, 2007–2017.
NOTE: In this figure, the "fentanyls" category includes fentanyl and fentanyl-related substances.

of the market, so in this section, we examine the DEA's public reports on its own seizures. Of course, the DEA does sometimes get involved in lower-level drug seizures, and there is no way to determine what share of these exhibits reflects retail versus wholesale markets, but one would expect these data to reflect, on average, larger samples and higher market levels than did the NFLIS data examined earlier because the DEA often focuses its efforts on importers and larger distributors.

Table 2.5 shows the number of DEA samples containing fentanyl (alone, with heroin, or with another drug) and other fentanyl-related novel synthetic opioids by year, from 2016 to 2018. As with all other indicators examined in this chapter, the counts increase over time, almost tripling over two years. Fentanyl retained a dominant share among the synthetic opioid seizures over all three years, and the shares in which it appeared with heroin or other drugs shifted, but not dramatically. Although not shown in Table 2.5, the mix of fentanyl analogs and other novel synthetic opioids changed over time and diversified. In 2016, the most-frequently reported fentanyl-related substances

Table 2.5
Synthetic Opioid Seizure Analysis from DEA Emerging Threat Reports

Opioid	Counts (Percentage)		
	2016	2017	2018
Fentanyl	877 (68)	1,873 (66)	2,723 (76)
Fentanyl only	408 (47)	805 (43)	1,062 (39)
Fentanyl and heroin	368 (42)	880 (47)	1,225 (45)
Fentanyl and other drugs	101 (12)	187 (10)	436 (16)
Fentanyl-related and novel synthetic opioids	422 (32)	952 (34)	868 (24)
Total	1,299	2,825	3,591

SOURCES: Data are from DEA Emerging Threat Reports (DEA, 2016a; DEA, 2017a; and DEA, 2018a).
NOTE: Percentages for the rows of fentanyl exhibits broken down by mixture are for the share of fentanyl seizures.

were furanyl fentanyl, acetyl fentanyl, and U-47700, in that order.[7] By 2018, the order was 4-ANPP (which is an immediate fentanyl precursor), acetyl fentanyl, and 4-fluoroisobutyryl fentanyl. Carfentanil and U-47700 exhibits increased from 2016 to 2017, but then sharply declined in 2018.

There is generally scant information about the purity of drug samples containing fentanyl, but the DEA's Fentanyl Signature Profiling Program (FSPP) analyzes a subset of drug seizures reported to the DEA as containing fentanyl, providing more quantitative measures. The DEA notes that these results are not intended to "reflect U.S. market share, but rather a snapshot of samples" submitted to the seven DEA laboratories (DEA, 2018b; DEA, 2019). Reports do not indicate where in the supply chain seizures were made (e.g., at retail or at wholesale). That said, most exhibits analyzed were of powders, with most being wholesale amounts (defined as 1 kg or more). FSPP did not include "seizures of very high purity fentanyl suspected as direct imports from China," suggesting that most of the seizures analyzed occurred after being smuggled into the United States (DEA, 2019).

Table 2.6 reports the breakdown of FSPP exhibits (separated by powders and tablets) for calendar years 2017 and 2018. The average purity for powder did not change over this short period (remaining steady at just more than 5 percent), but the figures ranged from 0.1 percent to almost 100 percent in both years. Retail-sized samples (less than 10 g) reported an average purity of just more than 2 percent in either year, which is similar to purity rates reported by international stakeholders (interviews can be found in Chapter Four). About three in ten powder exhibits contained heroin, which is slightly less than what was reported in the DEA's Emerging Threat Reports. Of those that contained heroin, the purity of both heroin and fentanyl declined, with the share of fentanyl declining at a greater rate, from 4.8 percent to 2.9 percent for fentanyl compared with 16.4 percent to 13 percent for heroin (DEA, 2018b; DEA, 2019).

---

[7] U-47700 is a potent illicit synthetic opioid. It is sometimes referred to as "pink" or "pinky."

Table 2.6
Breakdown of Fentanyl Seizures Reported in FSPP, 2017 and 2018

Fentanyl Seizures	Powders		Tablets	
	2017	2018	2017	2018
Total number of exhibits	692	568	72	100
Total weight	1,177 kg	723 kg	23 kg	112 kg
Fentanyl content	5.3%	5.2%	1.3 mg	1.5 mg
Range of fentanyl content	0.1–97.8%	0.1–96.8%	0.01–5.51 mg	0.02–4.84 mg
Share of seizures containing heroin	30%	32%	N/A	N/A
Number of retail exhibits (less than 10g)	72	34	N/A	N/A
Fentanyl content	2.5%	2.1%	N/A	N/A
Fentanyl-related exhibits	143	45	27	13

SOURCES: DEA, 2018d; DEA, 2019.
NOTES: A minor share of exhibits analyzed were neither tablet nor powder. There were eight liquid exhibits in 2017 and four tar exhibits in 2018. N/A = not applicable. Fentanyl-related exhibits are samples containing fentanyl analogs.

Pairing Laboratory Seizure Data with Fatal Synthetic Opioid Overdose Data

It is clear from our earlier discussion that the broad trends over time and across states in the overdose death and law enforcement data series have parallels. This section makes that explicit by juxtaposing some of those series graphically.

Figure 2.15 shows the upward trend in per capita counts of NFLIS seizures containing fentanyl and other analogs (red and blue bars, respectively) and the parallel rise in synthetic opioid overdose death rates reported by CDC and indexed to 100 percent in 2013 (green trend lines) for each U.S. Census division. (Each census region is divided into two or three "divisions.") The East North Central, New England, and Midatlantic divisions report sharp increases in NFLIS counts and almost tenfold increases in overdose deaths for synthetic

Figure 2.15
Per Capita NFLIS Counts for Fentanyl and Synthetic Opioid Overdose Death Rates, by Census Division

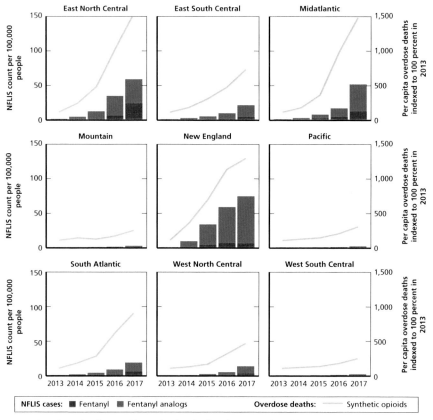

SOURCES: Seizure data (counts of fentanyl and analogs) are from NFLIS data tables, 2007 and 2017; overdose data are from deidentified MCOD certificate files produced by the National Center for Health Statistics and shared with RAND researchers under a data use agreement.
NOTES: Census divisions are each made up of a group of states. East North Central includes Illinois, Indiana, Michigan, Ohio, and Wisconsin. East South Central includes Alabama, Kentucky, Mississippi, and Tennessee. Midatlantic (or Middle Atlantic) includes New Jersey, New York, and Pennsylvania. Mountain includes Arizona, Colorado, Idaho, Montana, Nevada, New Mexico, Utah, and Wyoming. New England includes Connecticut, Maine, Massachusetts, New Hampshire, Rhode Island, and Vermont. Pacific includes Alaska, California, Hawaii, Oregon, and Washington. South Atlantic includes Delaware, the District of Columbia, Florida, Georgia, Maryland, North Carolina, South Carolina, Virginia, and West Virginia. West North Central includes Iowa, Kansas, Minnesota, Missouri, Nebraska, North Dakota, and South Dakota. West South Central includes Arkansas, Louisiana, Oklahoma, and Texas.

opioids by 2017. In contrast, the Mountain, Pacific, and West South Central divisions report smaller increases in NFLIS counts and slower rates of increase in overdose deaths.

That both NFLIS counts and overdose deaths rose and rose most sharply in the same divisions is apparent, but sometimes it is hard to judge how strong an association is when the growth is so rapid. Even in the hardest-hit divisions, the bars in 2013 and 2014 are very small. Thus, Figure 2.16 provides a scatter plot of the logged per capita rates of both series (after dropping state-year observations that contain zero seizures or deaths) and color codes the points by year. The fact that the upper right of the figure contains predominantly blue and purple dots shows that seizures and deaths have been rising over time. That there are some blue and purple dots in the middle or even lower-left of middle shows that some areas have not yet been severely affected.

Figure 2.16
Correlation Between Synthetic Opioid Overdoses and NFLIS Counts for Fentanyl

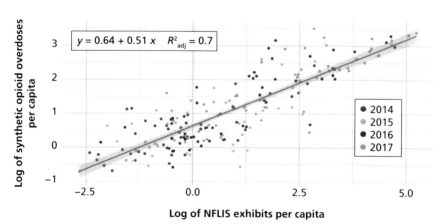

Log of NFLIS exhibits per capita

SOURCES: Seizure data (counts of fentanyl and analogs) are from NFLIS data tables, 2007 and 2017; overdose data are from deidentified MCOD certificate files produced by the National Center for Health Statistics and shared with RAND researchers under a data use agreement.
NOTES: The shading represents the pointwise 95-percent confidence interval around the linearly smoothed regression line. Number of observations = 202.
In the equation, y = log of synthetic opioid overdoses per capita, x = log of NFLIS fentanyl seizure counts per capita, and R^2 is a correlation coefficient.

The regression line passing through these points suggests that a 10-percent increase in NFLIS counts per 100,000 people is associated with a 5-percent increase in the per capita synthetic opioid overdose death rate. That is just an association, but the fact that most dots follow the line reasonably closely is a clear visual representation of the general agreement between the two very different data sources.

Summary of the Situation in the United States

Synthetic opioid overdoses and seizures increased dramatically between 2013 and 2017, yet remain concentrated in specific parts of the country, notably in Appalachia, the Midatlantic, and New England. Unsurprisingly, synthetic opioids are now involved in a substantial number of heroin overdose fatalities; dealers are known to mix fentanyls into heroin, presumably because they are so much cheaper per MED. What is perhaps more striking is that more than half of *cocaine* overdoses nationwide also include synthetic opioids, and those shares are much higher in such places as Ohio, West Virginia, and New England. It is still unclear how often such multidrug deaths are attributable to dealers intentionally or inadvertently mixing synthetic opioids into stimulants as opposed to users obtaining and ingesting the drugs together (e.g., goofballing or speedballing) or sequentially, but recent analysis of cocaine seizures in Ohio shows that fentanyl appeared in 12 percent of retail-level cocaine seizures.

Another striking observation is that, in some jurisdictions, the number of heroin overdose deaths is declining. That is not a surprise; it is consistent with the idea that more and more heroin dealers are supplementing their heroin with synthetic opioids. But if synthetic opioids were only being added to heroin, the total number of heroin overdoses should be rising with synthetic opioid overdoses. Instead, it appears that, in some markets, heroin is being replaced by—rather than merely supplemented with—more-potent opioids, such as fentanyl.

In some states, including some that have been hit hard, such as Massachusetts and New Hampshire, it is still fair to refer to a "fentanyl" problem. In other states, such as Ohio, seizure data reveal a wide variety of synthetic opioids, including extremely potent ones, such as carfentanil. This could be contributing to Ohio's disproportionately large number of overdoses. In 2017, more than 12 percent of synthetic opioid overdose deaths in the United States occurred in Ohio even though the state makes up less than 4 percent of the country's population.

The analysis—and its limitations—point to two concrete and feasible improvements that could be made to data reporting systems that would permit more-nuanced analysis. The first would be for the MCOD overdose data to report finer-grained distinctions among the synthetic opioids, instead of lumping all of them (except methadone) into a single ICD-10 code. Although textual analysis of death records shows that most overdoses in the past few years involved fentanyl (Hedegaard et al., 2018), that trend might not persist and better toxicological screens and data reporting on specific synthetic opioids could improve our understanding of changing market dynamics. Examination of overdose deaths using a single poisoning code is rather limiting.

Typical reporting on seizures distinguishes among the various synthetic opioids but reports only simple counts. That might have been adequate in the past, when a bag containing an illegal drug often contained just that drug. Now that there is a broad suite of opioids, not just heroin, and now that those opioids are showing up in packages of cocaine, it is important to start reporting counts of the various mixtures and combinations, not only total counts by chemical. Indeed, what would be better still would be to make available for analysis the underlying microdata so that adjustments could be made for purity and market level (as indicated by bag weight).

One key question is whether synthetic opioids will remain concentrated geographically or whether the hardest-hit states are bellwethers for what the nation as a whole might be confronting soon. And, if the latter, the question of which states in particular are the bellwethers remains, because close examination of states shows differences not only in the types of synthetic opioids but also in which drugs appear most often along with them in multiple-drug overdoses. Learning from these early exposure states could yield insights for public health and safety authorities.

CHAPTER THREE

Assessing Explanations for the Recent Rise in Synthetic Opioids

The arrival of fentanyl and other illicitly manufactured synthetic opioids caught most policymakers, scholars, and even users by surprise. Fentanyl was synthesized 60 years ago, so it is hardly a new substance, and some speculated long ago that it would supplant heroin as the dominant illicitly consumed opioid (Shulgin, 1975). Furthermore, as we discuss below, there were at least four nascent outbreaks in the United States in the past that failed to take root. This raises the question: Why now? More specifically, why is it that only in the past six years have some drug markets in North America witnessed a rapid and sustained transition toward illicitly manufactured fentanyl and novel synthetic opioids?

In this chapter, we examine the U.S. experience, drawing on research and policy analysis literature specific to synthetic opioids (in Chapter Four, we consider the experiences in other countries). We provide a brief history of fentanyl and its analogs, followed by an examination of some hypotheses regarding the arrival of these chemicals in drug markets in the United States. To ground the analysis, we examine earlier fentanyl outbreaks, comparing them with today's ongoing outbreak. This is followed by a review of a conceptual framework first proposed 25 years ago (Pickard, undated). We have compiled factors that fit into three conceptual themes, providing evidence for how, taken together, such factors contribute to today's problem.

Fentanyl: Dealer's Choice?

The answer to the question "Why did fentanyl emerge in 2013?" is not "Because it was invented in 2012." Rather, fentanyl was first synthesized in 1959 and introduced as an intravenous analgesic in Western Europe in 1963 (Stanley, 2014). After initial concern over its potency subsided, the U.S. Food and Drug Administration approved fentanyl as a general anesthetic in 1972 (Stanley, 2014; Vardanyan and Hruby, 2014). Its pharmacodynamics and ability to be synthesized from inexpensive and readily available chemical precursors instead of poppy made it a superior anesthetic to morphine (Suzuki and El-Haddad, 2017). Variations during synthesis can result in new analogs, some of which may have characteristics that are different from fentanyl (e.g., shorter duration of action, higher safety margin; Vardanyan and Hruby, 2014). Fentanyl analogs, such as sufentanil, alfentanil, remifentanil, and carfentanil, were developed not long after fentanyl itself for use in medical and veterinary settings (Armenian et al., 2018).

Although it was superior to traditional anesthetics, fentanyl's abuse potential was recognized. Early reports of misuse were limited to clinicians with ready access, such as anesthesiologists and surgeons (Armenian et al., 2018; Ward, Ward, and Saidman, 1983). Use of diverted fentanyl became a concern as the drug was reformulated in the 1990s into transdermal patches and lozenges to treat severe pain in palliative care for use outside of hospital settings (Armenian et al., 2018). Although uncommon, non-medical use of these pharmaceutical-grade sources of fentanyl continued into the early 2000s, with synthetic opioid overdose fatalities in the United States ranging from 800 to 1,600 per year (Hedegaard, Miniño, and Warner, 2018; Kramer and Tawney, 1998; Tharp, Winecker, and Winston, 2004). Although fentanyl and other synthetic opioids are used inappropriately, resulting in deaths, the staggering number of overdose fatalities involving synthetic opioids is believed to be the result of nonpharmaceutical (i.e., illicit) product sold as traditional street drugs, such as heroin and counterfeit prescription medications (DEA, 2018e; Gladden, Martinez, and Seth, 2016).

The most obvious explanation for why fentanyl and other synthetic opioids entered illicit markets has its roots in the United States' immense demand for opioids. Americans consume far more opioids for medical purposes than do citizens of any other country (both in absolute and per capita terms), and, traditionally, American consumption of illegal opioids (primarily heroin) has been substantial (International Narcotics Control Board, 2019; Musto, Korsmeyer, and Maulucci, 2002).

Some individuals who use drugs would seek better (i.e., more potent or purer) and cheaper forms of their favored products. All else being equal, fentanyl's higher potency compared with that of heroin should make it preferable, given its price. However, this assumes that individuals can distinguish (and might prefer) fentanyl's effects from those of other opioids available in illicit markets. The extent to which people who use drugs seek out more-potent synthetic opioids is unclear, although some report being able to distinguish its pharmacological effects from those of heroin (Mars, Rosenblum, and Ciccarone, 2018). Furthermore, dealers are not transparent when it comes to the distribution of synthetic opioids, using them to adulterate heroin or pressing them into tablets made to look like prescription medications (Baldwin et al., 2018; Ciccarone, Ondocsin, and Mars, 2017; DEA, 2018e). Fentanyl's arrival also has not been associated with increases in the numbers of opioid users, either in the United States or in other countries. Therefore, it is unlikely that the arrival of synthetic opioids stems from demand-side signals generated by consumers.

This leads us to consider supply. In this regard, Mars, Rosenblum, and Ciccarone (2018) discusses two broad supply-side explanations: (1) dealers reducing current costs or offsetting future costs and (2) supply shocks. The first explanation recognizes that DTOs are profit-maximizing businesses and that the low cost of synthetic opioids, especially relative to their morphine equivalence, makes them attractive alternatives to traditional illicit opioids, such as poppy-based heroin, which is susceptible to blight, drought, eradication, and labor shortages. Also, the very high potency-to-weight ratio of fentanyl and other synthetic opioids makes them easier to conceal and smuggle. Both of these factors matter insomuch as dealers seek to reduce their risks and the costs of doing business. Yet, these considerations were always present, and so by themselves cannot explain the sudden arrival of synthetic opioids in several drug markets around the world, starting around 2013.

Mars, Rosenblum, and Ciccarone (2018)'s second explanation, supply shocks, might better explain why a shift to synthetic opioids happens abruptly at a particular point in time.

Drug suppliers might turn to new products, such as synthetic opioids, as a response to constraints in their traditional supply chains brought on by poppy blights, crop eradication, or restrictions on their ability to access prescription opioids commonly diverted from loosely regulated pill mills or pharmacies. That theory, in part, fits Estonia, where fentanyl emerged at the same time that the Taliban's poppy ban disrupted heroin supplies in Europe (Mounteney et al., 2015). The North American version of this theory is that, as policies were enacted to reduce the prescribing of opioids for treating chronic pain, some individuals who had already developed opioid use disorder (OUD) began looking to illegal market alternatives, such as heroin (Alpert, Powell, and Pacula, 2017; Cicero, Ellis, and Surratt, 2012). Others might have transitioned simply because of tolerance developed from prescription pain relievers (Mars et al., 2014). Mars, Rosenblum, and Ciccarone (2018) posits that supply constraints in the licit and illicit markets, such as declines in poppy cultivation in Mexico around 2013, might have contributed to drug producers and dealers substituting fentanyl for heroin.

In theory, supply shocks could play some role in the substitution of fentanyl and the move away from heroin, but the heroin supply shock hypothesis does not account for a simultaneous transition toward fentanyl in illicit opioid markets in British Columbia, which were not and are not supplied by Mexican heroin (Ciccarone, 2009; Fischer et al., 2015) and which were not reported to experience a decrease in the availability of heroin (Ho et al., 2018). Nor is it entirely consistent with U.S. government and United Nations estimates, which show an expansion in Mexican heroin production between 2014 and 2017. Indeed, the 2016 estimate by the U.S. government is three times that for 2013 (ONDCP, 2018; United Nations Office on Drugs and Crime [UNODC], 2018).[1]

Mars, Rosenblum, and Ciccarone (2018) notes that fentanyl's arrival increased some individuals' preference for the drug because of its ability to overcome opioid tolerance (allowing some to again experience the euphoria associated with opioid use) and because of its lower cost in MEDs.[2] These are important considerations that could help explain fentanyl's staying power in drug markets. Yet, neither of these theories adequately explains the rapid transition witnessed across several drug markets in parts of Europe, Canada, and the United States. Instead, additional factors, some of which are specific to fentanyl, precipitated its widespread introduction to and circulation in contemporary illicit opioid markets. Understanding "why now" might help policymakers anticipate future developments, but to understand the current outbreak, it is necessary to examine earlier ones.

Previous Outbreaks and the Clandestine Production of Synthetic Opioids

Although the diversion of pharmaceutical fentanyl was documented at least as early as the 1980s and has persisted, there was little consideration of the possibility that illicitly manufactured fentanyl would enter drug markets as a substitute for heroin. However, at least one observer predicted exactly that. Forty years before the current crisis, chemist Alexander Shulgin predicted the rise of synthetic opioids, including fentanyl, in drug markets. According to Shulgin, "[t]he term 'when' rather than 'if' heroin substitutes appear is used intentionally, for this transformation seems economically inevitable" (Shulgin, 1975). Shulgin highlighted factors that would eventually drive this substitution,

---

[1]   Furthermore, there is disagreement about the direction of the recent trend in the purity-adjusted retail price for heroin in the United States (see Appendix B for more detail on this).

[2]   However, these cost savings might be reduced (or completely eliminated) because of the fact that fentanyl and several other synthetic opioids, which are more potent than heroin, have shorter durations of effects, necessitating more-frequent dosing.

including cheaper synthetic production and an ability to circumvent contemporary law enforcement efforts focused on eradicating poppy and interdicting heroin. Those are indeed compelling reasons, but they were just as compelling then as they are now.

The economic incentives that favor synthetic opioids over heroin are obvious, and fentanyl analogs began to appear in illicit markets as early as 1979, when "China White" was linked to 15 overdose deaths in suburban southern California (Henderson, 1988). These early outbreaks were initially thought to be the result of highly potent heroin but were later determined to be alpha-methylfentanyl and 3-methylfentanyl. At the time, those chemicals were not prohibited, but they were later added to Schedule I (the most restrictive drug category) by the DEA (Armenian et al., 2018). According to Henderson (1988), this was the first time clandestine laboratories were producing entirely new synthetic opioids as substitutes for heroin.

Throughout the 1980s, eight additional fentanyl analogs were identified in various heroin markets in California (Henderson, 1988). It is unclear how many individuals were involved in the manufacture and distribution of fentanyl analogs during this outbreak, but supply was largely restricted to markets in California and was linked to more than 100 fatal overdoses between 1979 and 1988 (Armenian et al., 2018; Henderson, 1988). Some suggest that these analogs were manufactured domestically by an individual or group trained in chemical synthesis (Henderson, 1988), although no source was discovered. The outbreaks in California eventually came to an end for reasons that are not altogether clear.

A second, independent outbreak occurred in the late 1980s, when a chemist at Calgon Carbon Corporation outside of Pittsburgh began producing 3-methylfentanyl, which was distributed to local drug markets. This outbreak resulted in dozens of overdoses, 18 of which were fatal (Hibbs, Perper, and Winek, 1991; Martin et al., 1991). Eventually, the chemist and several coconspirators were arrested, and the outbreak ended.

Another documented outbreak occurred between February 1991 and February 1993 in several regional drug markets on the East Coast, notably in Boston and New York. This outbreak, which resulted in

126 documented fatal overdoses, was linked to clandestine fentanyl and 3-methylfentanyl production in a remote laboratory in Wichita, Kansas (Coleman, 2007). Individuals involved in the distribution of the drug were suspected to have ties to organized crime in Boston (Mahony, 1993; Pickard, undated). A single highly skilled chemist was arrested, and the supply dried up.

The last documented and much larger outbreak in the United States prior to the current crisis occurred in several regional drug markets. Fentanyl mixed with heroin or cocaine arrived in street drug markets, resulting in about 1,000 fatal overdoses in Chicago, Detroit, and Philadelphia between April 2005 and March 2007 (CDC, 2008). In May 2006, Mexican law enforcement and the DEA identified and shut down the source, which was a clandestine laboratory in Toluca, Mexico (U.S. Department of Justice, National Drug Intelligence Center, 2006).[3] Fatal overdoses peaked the following month and then began declining, ending in early 2007 (CDC, 2008).

Table 3.1 shows these four documented fentanyl outbreaks, which were linked to clandestine production. There are some patterns. Three of the four are known to have involved a single chemist or lab and to have ended when that lab was shut down. To varying degrees, all of these outbreaks were localized geographically, and two of the larger outbreaks—in terms of the number of states covered and overdose deaths per year—were more recent and had known ties to organized criminal distribution networks.

These observations suggest that necessary conditions for a large and sustained outbreak might be: (1) production by multiple labs with ready access to precursor chemicals so that one successful enforcement

---

[3]   The chemist operating this lab, a Mexican national who immigrated to the United States as a child, previously served ten years in U.S. federal prison for illicit manufacture of fentanyl during the 1990s. He was deported in 2003 and soon started synthesizing fentanyl in Mexico for distribution to the United States (Coleman, 2007; Schaefer and Swickard, 2007). Some have speculated that the arrival of fentanyl in drug markets in and around Philadelphia during 2005 and 2006 was related to illicit opioid supply shocks, although the repatriation of a chemist with experience in illicit fentanyl manufacturing just prior to that outbreak might have been just as important (Hempstead and Yildirim, 2014; Mars, Rosenblum, and Ciccarone, 2018). In either case, the outbreak remained localized to several major markets and was short-lived.

Table 3.1
Four Previous Fentanyl Outbreaks

Place	Period	Confirmed Deaths	Synthetic Opioid	Source	Distribution Network	References
California	1979–1988, peak in 1984	112	Fentanyl and 3-methylfentanyl, alpha-methylfentanyl and eight other analogs sold as "China White" heroin	Unknown	Unclear, but deaths concentrated in California	Armenian et al. (2018); Henderson (1988)
Allegheny County, Pennsylvania	1988	18	3-methylfentanyl sold as "China White" heroin	Chemist at Calgon Carbon chemical company	Four other local conspirators arrested	"Synthetic Heroin Seen as Cause in 18 Deaths" (1988); Hibbs, Perper, and Wineck (1991); Martin et al. (1991)
Northeast, principally Boston and New York	1992–1993	126	Fentanyl and 3-methylfentanyl	Chemist in clandestine lab in Kansas	Organized crime in Boston	Coleman (2007); Pickard (undated)
Chicago, Detroit, and Philadelphia	2005–2007	1,013	Fentanyl	Chemist in clandestine lab in Mexico	Mexican DTO	Armenian et al. (2018); CDC (2008)

operation cannot shut down production, and (2) access to distribution capabilities, such as those organized crime has provided in the past for heroin and cocaine.

From the 1980s through the early 2000s, there were a large number of documented instances of clandestine fentanyl production in the United States that did not trigger outbreaks but had significant numbers of overdose deaths, often because there was no distribution network that could connect the supply to users. Sometimes production was by trained chemists (see Table 3.2). In two such instances, chemists at DuPont and the U.S. Naval Research Laboratory were arrested for synthesis of fentanyl analogs before ever distributing the drugs. In another instance, a self-trained chemist manufactured fentanyl in his home in Big Bear, California, using the internet to obtain synthesis instructions and locate potential buyers through chat rooms. In another instance, in 2005, the DEA dismantled a clandestine lab that was synthesizing and pressing fentanyl powder into counterfeit oxycodone tablets. Internet distribution and the counterfeiting of prescription tablets both returned in the current outbreak.

The common denominators in the cases of the stillborn epidemics described in Table 3.2 are single points of production and/or limited distribution capability.

The Current Outbreak

Much of today's fentanyl and related substances originate in China. According to federal law enforcement, these substances arrive in U.S. markets directly from Chinese manufacturers in cargo or via the post or private parcel service (e.g., UPS, FedEx), smuggled from Mexico, or smuggled from Canada after being pressed into counterfeit prescription pills (O'Connor, 2017; ONDCP, 2017). It is not known what shares of fentanyl and related substances are supplied by what country and route, although the DEA suggests that some portion of fentanyl is produced in Mexico using precursors from China (DEA, 2017b).

Seizures of fentanyl imports have increased in the past few years. CBP reports that the bulk weight of fentanyl seizures has increased

Table 3.2
Seizures of Domestic Clandestine Fentanyl Production

Place	Period of Operation	Synthetic Opioid	Source	Distribution Network	References
Delaware	1985	3-methylfentanyl	Chemist at DuPont chemical company	None, producer arrested	Henderson (1988)
Washington, D.C.	1986	3-methylfentanyl	Chemist at U.S. Naval Research Laboratory	None, producer arrested	Coleman (2007); Pickard (undated)
San Jose, California	1990	Fentanyl	Clandestine lab	Unknown	U.S. Department of Justice, National Drug Intelligence Center (2006)
San Diego, California	1990–1991	Fentanyl	Chemists in clandestine labs; one chemist later deported to Mexico where he started operations in 2005	Local network; six other conspirators arrested	Coleman (2007); Omphroy (1992)
Fallbrook, California	1991	Fentanyl	Clandestine lab	Unknown	U.S. Department of Justice, National Drug Intelligence Center (2006)

Table 3.2—Continued

Place	Period of Operation	Synthetic Opioid	Source	Distribution Network	References
Big Bear, California	2000	Fentanyl	Self-taught chemist using techniques from the internet in a clandestine lab	Producer used internet chatrooms to find buyers	U.S. Department of Justice, National Drug Intelligence Center (2006); Smith (2001)
Newtown Square, Pennsylvania	2003	Fentanyl	Clandestine lab	Unknown	U.S. Department of Justice, National Drug Intelligence Center (2006); Parker (2006)
Santa Clara, California	2004	Fentanyl	Clandestine lab	Unknown	U.S. Department of Justice, National Drug Intelligence Center (2006)
San Diego, California	2005	Fentanyl	Clandestine lab	Unknown	U.S. Department of Justice, National Drug Intelligence Center (2006)
Azusa, California	2005	Fentanyl	Clandestine lab pressing fentanyl into counterfeit oxycodone tablets	Unknown	U.S. Department of Justice, National Drug Intelligence Center (2006)

from near zero (1 kg) in 2013 to almost a metric ton in FY 2018 (CBP, 2019a). Seizures of fentanyl shipped by post also have increased. From late 2014 until the beginning of 2017, the U.S. Postal Inspection Service seized about 100 parcels that contained synthetic opioids (ONDCP, 2017). By FY 2017, postal seizures had increased to more than 220 events that year (CBP, 2018). As of FY 2018, postal seizures had doubled to 455 events (CBP, 2019a). Increases in seizures could reflect greater law enforcement efforts.

According to authorities, the purity of postal seizures originating in China is upward of 90 percent, while the product seized on the border with Mexico is typically 5- to 10-percent pure (DEA, 2017b; ONDCP, 2017). Adjusting for purity between seizures at mail and express consignment facilities and those at land ports of entry suggests that the majority of purity-adjusted fentanyl seized is arriving from China (Pardo, 2018).

Today's epidemic includes more than just fentanyl. According to forensic laboratory data, the number of novel synthetic opioids, many of which have not been seen before, is growing, as is the number of extremely potent analogs, such as carfentanil (Pardo, Davis, and Moore, forthcoming). The ongoing outbreak has heavily affected a substantial part of the country, rather than being localized to a single market, and the areas affected are increasing each year. Table 3.3 compares today's crisis with prior outbreaks.

Factors That Contribute to the Rise of Fentanyl and Other Synthetic Opioids Today

The demand for opioids in the United States and the disruption of the supply of traditionally used opioids might have contributed to fentanyl's rise. Yet the sudden and expansive arrival of synthetic opioids across illicit markets in various countries points to additional supply-side factors, some of which are specific to these chemicals. Here we draw from a 1996 presentation made by William Pickard titled "Factors Promoting the Spread of Fentanyl Manufacture" (Pickard, 1996). We have modified and added to his original list, arriving at seven factors that

Table 3.3
Comparing U.S. Fentanyl Outbreaks

Aspect	Prior Outbreaks	Today's Outbreak
Location	Generally localized	Not localized, although there is regional variation
Duration	Generally short; only one lasted more than two years	Nearly six years
Chemicals	Fewer analogs; no reports of super-potent opioids (e.g., carfentanil)	Fentanyl dominates, but there are many analogs and super-potent opioids
Source	Often labs in the United States, with one exception	Almost all is imported, mostly from China and Mexico
Distribution	Limited, although two employed traditional illicit market actors	More widespread; both traditional illicit market actors and mail order or internet
Sold as	Often heroin, although some noted it showing up in cocaine	Heroin and prescription pills, but an increasing share of cocaine and psychostimulant overdoses mention synthetic opioids

we group into three themes: chemical, regulatory, and technological and economic.

We note that several factors could belong to more than one of the themes (for example, design of new fentanyl analogs is directly related to regulatory decisions to control emerging substances; Armenian et al., 2018). Therefore, these factors and their overarching themes should not be thought of as fully independent of each other when considering fentanyl's rise. These categories and factors are

- chemical
    - diffusion of simpler and more-efficient synthesis methods
    - a move from chemists to cooks
    - design of analogs
- regulatory
    - lack of effective precursor controls and industry oversight
- technological and economic
    - expanding distribution networks
    - reduced smuggling risks and increased licit trade
    - preexisting market conditions.

These factors provide a useful framework for understanding fentanyl's sudden rise and the continued generation of novel synthetic opioids, which, like other novel psychoactives, are often found to enter and exit illicit markets (Pardo, Davis, and Moore, forthcoming; Reuter and Pardo, 2017). Several of these factors, such as the lack of precursor controls or generation of simpler synthesis methods, were already in place before the 2013 rise of fentanyl—sometimes for quite some time, making it impossible to point to any one as the sole cause of fentanyl's rise. Yet, taken together, they offer a possible explanation as to why this current outbreak is more geographically diffuse, chemically varied, harmful, and sustained over time.

We do not discuss the seventh factor—preexisting market conditions—because this consideration is largely related to the demand for opioids and potential supply shocks discussed earlier. These are important conditions that can contribute to the rise of fentanyl in a market. To our knowledge, fentanyl has not arrived in jurisdictions without an established opioid user population.

Chemical
Diffusion of Simpler and More-Efficient Synthesis Methods
Pickard notes that online dissemination of new "cookbook" methods will promote fentanyl's spread (Pickard, 1996). This refers to both the accessibility of synthesis methods made possible by the internet and the generation of easier-to-follow and more procedurally simple synthesis methods that do not require the use of dangerous intermediate chemicals or expensive precursors. In some instances, these easier and less dangerous synthesis techniques can be used outside the laboratory and without sophisticated or specialized equipment. Several of these techniques support the ability to synthesize fentanyl at room temperature.

Innovations in synthesis methods often result in higher yields with fewer steps (e.g., sometimes combining reactions or modifying certain intermediate steps to reduce time and inputs). Some new synthesis methods employ common chemical inputs, obviating the need for costlier chemicals. Increasing yield (i.e., the amount remaining after chemical reactions) minimizes the amount lost in the result of the reactions. As noted in several articles in the literature, purification will result in lower yields but purer product (Gupta et al., 2005). There-fore, increasing yields and cutting the number of reaction steps can reduce waste and the labor and time required to produce final product, and may eliminate the need for dangerous or hard to obtain chemi-cal inputs. The logical implication is that more-efficient and simpler synthesis methods in turn facilitate production and help conceal the footprint and waste generated by labs that do not want to attract the attention of authorities.

Synthesis methods for fentanyl can sometimes be modified by combining steps from other synthesis routes (Mayer et al., 2016). This is sometimes done to optimize the procedure or utilize alternative intermediate chemicals or pre-precursors. In either case, the increase and diffusion of fentanyl synthesis routes might make manufacture accessible to chemists with modest skills while also providing innova-tive chemists with ideas for further optimization or utilization of alter-native chemicals.

Table 3.4 summarizes the often-cited articles in the English-language fentanyl synthesis literature. Although we include several articles published by Chinese and Taiwanese research chemists, our analysis fails to capture other non–English-language sources on syn-thesis methods. For brevity, we have omitted many other articles cited in the published and patent literature relevant to the synthesis of other analogs—including carfentanil—that might offer additional improve-ments or insights for fentanyl synthesis (Malaquin et al., 2010; Váradi et al., 2015).

Paul Janssen published his fentanyl synthesis methods in the early 1960s (Janssen, 1961; Janssen and Eddy, 1960). This synthesis route starts with N-benzyl-4-piperidone and is often considered a difficult route that requires maintaining controlled conditions and high tem-peratures while using dangerous solvents to produce fentanyl in modest yields (Hsu and Banks, 1992; Yadav et al., 2010). The DEA suggests that such a synthesis method is "beyond the rudimentary skills of most clandestine" chemists and that "only individuals who have acquired advanced chemistry knowledge and skills have successfully used this synthesis route" (21 CFR Part 1310, 2007).

Table 3.4
Fentanyl Synthesis Literature

Publication	Steps	Overall Yield	Comments
Janssen (1961)	5	No yield mentioned	Uses caustic reagents, requires controlled environment, and is time-consuming. High level of skills required
Zee, Lai, and Wu (1981)	6	< 41%	Use of different precursors to reduce costs (instead of 1-benzyl-4-piperidone)
Jonczyk et al. (1978)	5	< 40%	Use of different intermediate chemicals. Requires controlled environment and use of caustic chemicals
Zong, Yin, and Ji (1979)	5	< 35%	—
Zee and Wang (1980)	5	< 30%	Novel method to derive fentanyl from pyridine
Hsu and Banks (1992)	6	85–90%	Improves on Zee et al. (1981). Can synthesize preceding compounds in higher yields, isolating fentanyl in the last step in the same pot
Suh, Cho, and Shin (1998)	4	33%	—
Siegfried (undated)	4	50–80%	Uses NPP. Simple procedure that does not require controlled environment
Gupta et al. (2005)	3	40%	One-pot synthesis, can be done at room temperature
Fu et al. (2011)	3	45%	Efficient synthesis of intermediate chemicals to yield highly pure fentanyl using simple starting materials under mild conditions
Gaffarzadeh, Joghan, and Faraji (2012)	2	84%	Novel synthesis of amides, but requires additional chemical agents

Table 3.4—Continued

Publication	Steps	Overall Yield	Comments
Gupta et al. (2013)	4	65%	Novel synthesis of analogs, but uses caustic chemicals
Valdez, Leif, and Mayer (2014)	3	73–78%	Discusses synthesis of several analogs. Very efficient method; it combines several steps used by other synthesis methods
Walz and Hsu (2017)	4	53%	Starts with 1-benzyl-4-piperidone but employs more-efficient purification methods

NOTE: Several of these synthesis articles are affiliated with a national defense research institute in the United States, India, or China.

Since Janssen's methods were published, alternative synthesis routes have been published in the scientific literature to increase yields while reducing the number of steps and the use of harmful, expensive, or difficult-to-obtain chemicals. From the late 1970s to the early 1990s, several methods were published with the goal of enhancing supply for legitimate use (Hsu and Banks, 1992; Jonczyk et al., 1978; Zee and Wang, 1980; Zee, Lai, and Wu, 1981).

However, some had intended to promote the synthesis of fentanyl for illegitimate purposes. One synthesis method, written under a pseudonym, appeared freely online in the 1990s and provided an important advance. This method—the Siegfried method—improved on alternative synthesis routes published during the 1980s, starting with commercially available N-phenethyl-4-piperidone (NPP) (21 CFR Part 1310, 2007; Siegfried, undated; Yadav et al., 2010). This method, which was published explicitly for illicit manufacture (the author even included steps so that dealers could dilute product for retail distribution), was simple, did not require special equipment or the use of dangerous chemicals, and could yield a high amount of fentanyl (Yadav et al., 2010). It also offered steps for synthesis of several analogs by modifying intermediate chemicals. This synthesis method appealed to at-home chemists. Of the five domestic clandestine fentanyl laboratories seized by the DEA between 2000 and 2005, four employed this route (21 CFR Part 1310, 2007). The Siegfried method was also suspected to be the method employed in the laboratory in Toluca, Mexico, which was shut down by the DEA and Mexican law enforcement in 2006 (Coleman, 2007).

After the Siegfried method was published online, several other synthesis routes entered the research literature. Most of these also use NPP. Several of these methods have titles that mention "convenient," "optimized," or "operationally simple" synthesis routes. Gupta et al. (2005) proposes a "one pot" method that synthesizes fentanyl in a simple and efficient manner under nonlaboratory conditions at room temperature. The article omits separation and purification steps, which would increase purity while reducing yield.

Since Gupta et al.'s (2005) one-pot method was published, other articles have been published examining novel or more-efficient synthesis routes, including the synthesis of several fentanyl analogs (Fu et al., 2011; Ghaffarzadeh, Joghan, and Faraji, 2012; Gupta et al., 2013). Ghaffarzadeh, Joghan, and Faraji (2012) details operationally simple synthesis steps that generate good yields under mild reaction conditions and short reaction times. Fu et al.'s synthesis method claims to have decent overall yields of highly pure fentanyl starting with simple materials (Fu et al., 2011).

Research into simplifications in fentanyl synthesis continued to be published during the first years of the current outbreak. In late 2014, Valdez and colleagues published an open-access article on the synthesis of fentanyl and several analogs using a three-step route optimized to produce high yields (Valdez, Leif, and Mayer, 2014). This route improves synthesis by combining several intermediate steps. As of March 2019, according to the open-access publisher that tracks viewer metrics, the manuscript has been downloaded more than 70,000 times. In the first year of publication, it was downloaded, on average, less than 200 times per month. By the end of its fourth year in publication, it boasted more than 3,000 downloads per month.

Advances in novel synthesis methods continue. In 2017, several years into the current outbreak, Walz and Hsu published an additional synthesis technique starting with N-benzyl-4-piperidone but employing more-efficient purification methods based on their earlier work improving the synthesis of intermediates in the production of carfentanil, sufentanil, and remifentanil (Walz and Hsu, 2017).

Although several simplified synthesis methods have been published in the past few years, federal law enforcement documents note only the Siegfried and Janssen methods (DEA, 2018b). However, it is not entirely clear to what extent other synthesis routes are used in fentanyl production, given existing signature analysis methods.[4] DEA chemists note two fentanyl synthesis profiling methods (Casale, Mallette, and Guest, 2017; Lurie et al., 2012), which focus on "manufacturing impurities that are unique to [the Janssen or Siegfried] synthetic routes" (Lurie et al., 2012, p. 191). However, other sources note

---

[4] A similar phenomenon is noted in the DEA's heroin signature program, which for years mistakenly attributed Mexican powdered heroin to Colombian origins (DEA, 2018c).

that clandestine operators are likely to use routes that start with NPP, such as the one-pot method by Gupta et al. (2005) and the Valdez method (Valdez, Leif, and Mayer, 2014; Mayer et al., 2016). To enhance fentanyl synthesis attribution, analytical chemists at Lawrence Livermore Laboratories, building off of the work of Lurie and colleagues (2012), state that "[f]orensic chemical attribution of synthetic schemes that rely on a common intermediate . . . are often difficult to discriminate amongst due to a small number of unique signatures, particularly when present at trace levels" (Mayer et al., 2016). Therefore, the extent to which the Janssen or Siegfried methods are currently employed by clandestine manufactures (as opposed to the other synthesis methods discussed earlier) is unclear.

Several of the aforementioned articles mention that analogs can be synthesized by adapting fentanyl's synthesis method with minor variation in inputs or steps. More-recent synthesis methods in the literature report increased yields or reductions in the number of steps. Except for Walz and Hsu (2017), most of the recent synthesis methods use NPP, a similar derivative, or its commercially available precursors (i.e., fentanyl pre-precursors). Some discuss optimized synthesis or purification methods, offering simpler and more-efficient production. These articles are often available online, sometimes with free, open access. Several discuss the use of alternative or less dangerous chemicals, making synthesis more accessible to those without advanced chemistry degrees or those lacking access to inputs or equipment.

Move from Chemists to Cooks

The invention and dissemination of easier synthesis methods can render a much broader set of individuals qualified and capable of producing fentanyl. Pickard (1996) notes that a move from a few skilled individuals to "many untrained groups" will increase fentanyl manufacturing. Many early outbreaks were limited, in part because producers were often highly trained chemists; some worked at well-known chemical companies or military research establishments. Arresting a single chemist successfully interrupted clandestine production because that skilled individual was hard to replace. The DEA has noted that the Siegfried method is favored by at-home chemists (21 CFR Part 1310,

2008). Other methods mentioned earlier offer straightforward synthesis techniques in a single vessel at room temperature.

The scale of China's underregulated industries allows for minimally trained technicians with access to the proper inputs to follow simple synthesis steps while avoiding oversight. China's pharmaceutical and industrial chemical industries are large and beyond the reach of U.S. law enforcement. The number of active pharmaceutical ingredient manufacturers in China is estimated to be about 5,000, while there might be up to 400,000 chemical manufacturers and distributors (O'Connor, 2017).[5] In many ways, production of fentanyl and novel synthetic opioids stems from the larger phenomenon of novel psychoactive substances. Europe has witnessed the rise of uncontrolled psychoactives, mostly synthetic cannabinoids and cathinones arriving from China, for about a decade and half (EMCDDA, 2018b).

The move to minimally trained cooks is also reported elsewhere. Since late 2017, four rudimentary clandestine labs, some with ties to organized crime, have been shut down in Mexico. Three were in densely populated residential areas in major cities, such as Mexicali and Mexico City ("PGR Asegura Supuesto Laboratorio de Fentanilo en CDMX," 2018; DEA, 2018e; "Aseguran en Culiacán, Sinaloa presunto laboratorio de fentanilo," 2019; La Procuraduría General de la República, 2017; "Médico búlgaro, exmilitar, Kulkin tenía, en un cuartito de Mexicali, laboratorio 'AAA' de fentanilo," 2018). Largely gone are the days of a single highly-trained chemist synthesizing fentanyl in a professional laboratory. The potential scale of chemical and pharmaceutical manufacturing, especially in China, combined with more-accessible synthesis techniques allows for the untrained to manufacture fentanyl virtually anywhere, making supply disruption more challenging.

---

[5] The U.S. State Department's 2015 International Narcotics Control Strategy Report (INCSR) notes that there are "400,000 chemical distributors or suppliers in China" (U.S. State Department, 2015), although the 2014 INCSR notes that there are approximately 160,000 "precursor chemical companies" (U.S. State Department, 2014).

Design of Analogs

Design of analogs relates to the diffusion of novel synthesis methods and precursor controls but also is driven by decisions by the DEA to place certain chemicals on the list (or schedule) of controlled (i.e., prohibited) substances (Reuter and Pardo, 2017). It does not explain fentanyl's sudden rise, but placing one chemical on the schedule of controlled substances might contribute to the rise of another very similar but not-yet-scheduled substance (i.e., an analog; Armenian et al., 2018). Novel synthesis methods detail variations in fentanyl manufacture that can be used to develop such analogs. Furthermore, the control of such precursors as NPP might encourage some producers to adopt alternatives, which could generate new analogs in the process.

Online vendors in China appear to respond to the scheduling of one chemical by supplying new analogs that are not yet prohibited (Pardo, Davis, and Moore, forthcoming; U.S. Senate, Permanent Subcommittee on Investigations, Committee on Homeland Security and Governmental Affairs, 2018). As discussed in Chapter Two, domestic seizure data in the United States reported to NFLIS show a dramatic increase in novel synthetic opioids and fentanyl analogs. Likewise, the number of novel synthetic opioids reported in early warning systems both in Europe and globally has increased in recent years, from four in 2012 to 46 in 2017 (EMCDDA, 2018b; UNODC, 2019).

This has led the DEA to emergency schedule all substances "structurally related to fentanyl," effectively placing a generic control on the entire family of fentanyl chemicals (DEA, 2018b). At the request of the United States, China has adopted a similar generic control on all fentanyl-related chemicals, although the results of this step remain to be seen (Liu, 2019).

Generic controls on fentanyl might deter some manufacturers from developing new analogs that are structurally similar to fentanyl, but novel synthetic opioids, such as the Upjohn (e.g., U-47700) and Allen and Hanburys (e.g., AH-7921) series, are not structurally related to fentanyl. Many of these drugs were synthesized decades ago as potential medications but are now emerging as drugs that are sold online (Katselou et al., 2015; Solimini et al., 2018). The research literature details the synthesis methods of these and other novel synthetic opioids (Solimini et al., 2018; World Health Organization [WHO], 2014). Efforts to curb the fentanyl supply might be stymied by the development and dissemination of synthesis methods for other novel synthetic opioids.

Regulatory
Lack of Effective Precursor Controls and General Regulatory Oversight

The lack of domestic and international controls on precursors is mentioned by Pickard (1996) as a contributing factor to the rise of fentanyl. Although there are several fentanyl precursors, much of the synthesis literature describes the use of two precursors: NPP and 4-ANPP. After the 2005–2007 fentanyl outbreak in the United States, the DEA controlled NPP and 4-ANPP under federal law (21 CFR Part 1310, 2007; 21 CFR Part 1310, 2008). However, NPP and 4-ANPP were not subject to United Nations drug control conventions until October 2017 (International Narcotics Control Board, 2017). Before that, there were no import or export reporting requirements or restrictions, and no country was obligated to apply internal regulatory oversight on the domestic production or trade of such precursors. These two chemicals were brought into control in Mexico in July 2017 and in China in February 2018 (DEA, 2018d; Secretariat of the Interior, 2017).

China, in particular, still lacks the necessary enforcement and oversight capacity to regulate its massive pharmaceutical and chemical industries (Pardo, 2018; Pardo, Kilmer, and Huang, 2019). It remains to be seen whether these precursor controls will reduce or limit synthesis of fentanyl using NPP or 4-ANPP. It is possible that producers might move to other uncontrolled precursors. In fact, 1-benzyl-4-piperidone, which was first used by Janssen in fentanyl synthesis, is not subject to control in the United States or internationally. Likewise, other precursors are used in the synthesis of fentanyl analogs. For example, 3-methylfentanyl can be synthesized from 3-methyl-N-phenethylpiperidin-4-one (3MNPP).

Developing a comprehensive set of precursor controls is a substantial challenge, given the many alternative methods for synthesizing fentanyl analogs and the use of common organic pre-precursors, such as 4-piperidinone and phenethylamine (Hsu and Banks, 1992). It is possible that producers could quickly adapt by using alternative precursors or synthesis methods that avoid starting with NPP or 4-ANPP.

Technological and Economic
Expanding Distribution Networks

Previous fentanyl outbreaks were limited in part because producers often did not have the means to distribute product. In several cases, law enforcement arrested producers before they could sell fentanyl (Coleman, 2007; Henderson, 1988). By contrast, the deadlier outbreaks described in Table 3.2 were linked to criminal distribution networks, allowing product to enter illicit drug markets, often disguised as a more-potent form of heroin. The outbreak in the early 1990s was associated with organized crime in the Northeast and the 2005–2007 outbreak was linked to Mexican drug traffickers.

As mentioned earlier, law enforcement notes two sources for illicit fentanyl and related substances. Mexican DTOs are linked to fentanyl smuggling and distribution (DEA, 2018e). However, technological advances in communication and trade in the past decade have given producers access to an alternate structure of distribution networks via the internet (Aldridge and Décary-Hétu, 2016).

Unlike dark web marketplaces, which require knowledge of advanced routing software and access to cryptocurrency, surface web vendors, often located in Asia, can be found easily from a simple internet search. Many of these vendors claim to ship product directly to buyers anywhere in the world and accept various forms of payment, including cryptocurrency, money orders, and wire transfers (U.S. Senate, Permanent Subcommittee on Investigations, Committee on Homeland Security and Governmental Affairs, 2018; Pardo, Davis, and Moore, forthcoming). In one recent analysis of eight easy-to-find fentanyl vendors from overseas, almost all had domain registries that were purchased in the past three years; the oldest was registered in early 2014 (Pardo, Davis, and Moore, forthcoming). There have been reports of individuals purchasing fentanyl from manufacturers in China for distribution downstream, sometimes using dark web marketplaces to reach end users online (U.S. Department of Justice, 2018).

The ability of enterprising drug dealers to obtain fentanyl and other related substances without leaving the comfort of their homes reduces barriers to market entry. Importantly, this obviates the need to interact with violent criminal organizations that smuggle drugs across international borders. Access via the internet and mail link manufacturers and buyers even when they are thousands of miles apart, diminishing the risks and costs associated with smuggling the drug. This reduction in barriers might encourage some dealers to adopt fentanyl before traditional heroin sources are interrupted or attract some individuals to drug distribution without the need to engage potentially violent criminal actors.

Fentanyl's potency and low cost of production allow for convenient and operationally simple distribution via the postal system. In such cases, enterprising individuals living in economically depressed areas where opioid use is endemic might see an opportunity to enter drug distribution to supplement their income (MacCoun and Reuter, 1992).

Reduced Smuggling Risks and Expanded Licit Trade

Fentanyl's potency-to-weight ratio makes it ideal for smuggling. A small amount of fentanyl can be easily concealed through traditional conveyances, packed in vehicles or hidden on the person. The supply of minute amounts of fentanyl through mail and private package services is profitable to someone who can redistribute it to local markets; even an ounce of fentanyl can substitute for 1 kg of heroin.[6] What is different is the rise in the volume of mail arriving from China and the wider adoption of cryptocurrency—such as BitCoin—and software—such as The Onion Router (TOR)—that safeguard online anonymity (Crosby et al., 2016; Martin, 2014; U.S. Senate, Permanent Subcommittee on Investigations, Committee on Homeland Security and Governmental Affairs, 2018).

Rising e-commerce and the growth of inbound packages from China overlap with fentanyl's arrival. In 2011, postal services of the

---

[6] In addition, it is plausible that the replacement cost of the drug at the point of seizure is likely to be negatively correlated with the seizure rate. Smugglers are likely to invest more to prevent interdiction of more-valuable shipments.

United States and China entered into an agreement to streamline mail delivery and reduce shipping costs for merchandise originating in China (U.S. Postal Service [USPS], 2011). This "ePacket" service is designed for shipping consumer goods (under 2 kg) from China directly and rapidly to customers ordering items online (U.S. Senate, Permanent Subcommittee on Investigations, Committee on Homeland Security and Governmental Affairs, 2018; USPS, 2011). Before the advent of ePackets, items mailed from China would take more than a month to arrive, unless one opted for more-expensive private couriers (Moshin, 2018). Fast and affordable shipping of manufactured goods from China has increased inbound package volume. In FY 2012, USPS handled about 27 million ePackets from China (USPS, 2014). This increased to nearly 500 million ePackets by 2017 (U.S. Senate, Permanent Subcommittee on Investigations, Committee on Homeland Security and Governmental Affairs, 2018). This figure does not include items from China arriving by cargo or private consignment operators, such as DHL or FedEx.

For reference, if the total U.S. heroin market was on the order of 45 pure metric tons (45,000 kg; Midgette et al., 2019) before fentanyl and if fentanyl is 25 times more potent than heroin, then it would only take 1,800 1-kg parcels to supply the same amount of MEDs to meet the demand for the entire U.S. heroin market.

Today, shipping costs from China are negligible. A 1-kg parcel can be shipped from China to the United States for as little as $10 through the international postal system or for $100 by private consignment operator (Pardo, Davis, and Moore, forthcoming). The volume of mail and cargo from China gives adequate cover for smuggling minute quantities of fentanyl or other novel synthetic opioids. Online vendors realize this and often prefer sending packages through USPS, sometimes targeting processing centers that handle large volumes of mail (Pardo, Davis, and Moore, forthcoming).

The Rise of Fentanyl

Illicitly manufactured synthetic opioids entering U.S. drug markets have been documented several times since the late 1970s. These early outbreaks were generally localized and short-lived. Although a few observers had foreshadowed fentanyl eclipsing heroin, rarely did it persist or expand outside these nascent outbreaks. The extent to which early outbreaks were related to specifically timed economic events that might have encouraged substitution is unclear. During earlier outbreaks, production was limited to a few capable chemists, but bottlenecks in production and challenges in distribution slowed fentanyl's diffusion.

Some experts speculate that recent shocks in the heroin supply largely contributed to fentanyl's rise. We are skeptical that this factor alone can explain the rise of synthetic opioids, given that fentanyl has simultaneously appeared in Canada and in parts of Europe that have not experienced heroin supply shocks (see Appendix B). Rather, we believe that a confluence of factors explains such a phenomenon. Some of these factors are specific to fentanyl, while others helped facilitate its spread. In many ways, fentanyl's rise is another chapter in the saga of new psychoactive substances produced overseas for developed drug markets.

The rediscovery and manufacture of novel synthetic opioids is aided by advances in the dissemination of novel, easier, and more-efficient synthesis methods, some of which detail synthesis routes for several fentanyl analogs. Growing e-commerce and the advent of other innovations meant to enhance online privacy (e.g., BitCoin, TOR browsing) make online trade in these substances attractive. These operational shifts have expanded the once-limited fentanyl distribution networks, making these substances accessible to anyone with an internet connection and an address to redistribute them in illicit markets.

Compounding all this is poor regulatory oversight in China and easier access to precursor chemicals. China's large and underregulated pharmaceutical and chemical industries create opportunities for anyone with access to the inputs to synthesize fentanyl or manufacture precursors. Mexican DTOs, which have a history of importing methamphetamine precursors from China, are now importing fentanyl precursors (O'Connor, 2016). Today, illicit fentanyl is no longer manufactured by a single producer in a clandestine laboratory.

China's economy, particularly its pharmaceutical and chemical industries, have grown at levels that outpace regulatory oversight, allowing suppliers to avoid regulatory scrutiny and U.S. law enforcement (O'Connor, 2017; Pardo, 2018). Likewise, rising trade and e-commerce originating in China since 2011 facilitate the diffusion of potent synthetic opioids. Drug distribution has been further facilitated by the advent of cryptocurrencies and anonymous browsing software.

As Shulgin stated almost 45 years ago, fentanyl's arrival was a question of "when" and not "if" (Shulgin, 1975). Several outbreaks have occurred over the years, but they ended once the source was found and producers were arrested. It was only a matter of time before these factors aligned, resulting in cheap and mass-produced synthetic opioids. Individuals and companies in China, which boasts both large and underregulated industries and many individuals with knowledge of chemical synthesis, are contributing to a massive influx of synthetic opioids into North America that is complicating traditional supply-side efforts.

CHAPTER FOUR

International Experiences with Synthetic Opioids

Although fentanyl and its analogs have caused more deaths in the United States than they have in any other nation, the United States is not the only country to experience problems with these substances. As of this writing, Canada is suffering a comparably severe problem. Estonia, a very small country (of 1.3 million inhabitants) that neighbors Russia, has had a serious fentanyl problem for almost 20 years. A few other northern European countries have experienced problems with fentanyl or with other synthetic opioids; sometimes these problems are associated with supply shocks in the preexisting illegal opioid market. In this chapter, we describe commonalities and differences in how fentanyl and related substances are affecting other countries to address the following questions:

- What are the characteristics of fentanyl markets in other countries?
- How have these markets evolved?
- What are the notable commonalities and areas of divergence across these markets?
- What insights do these countries' experiences offer for U.S. policymakers and researchers?

As discussed in Chapter One, this chapter draws primarily on a review of literature and official documentation from the focus countries and on interviews with key informants who were in positions to comment on drug markets in their respective countries (or more

broadly). Further detail on these stakeholder interviews is provided in Appendix E.

After explaining how countries were selected, we provide a historical overview and description of national market characteristics, followed by a discussion of the user population and drug-related harms, and a brief summary of the current situation in each country. Subsequently, we compare market characteristics and identify possible factors associated with the emergence of fentanyl and related substances. Finally, we discuss emerging themes and lessons for the United States.

Selection of Focus Countries

In this chapter, we examine five countries and offer a variety of contexts for the emergence of fentanyl. Specifically, we focus on

- countries with a long-term fentanyl presence: Currently, **Estonia** is the only such country
- countries experiencing a recent emergence of fentanyl—specifically, **Canada, Latvia,** and **Sweden**
- countries with a conspicuous absence of fentanyl: **Finland** has a unique opioid market largely devoid of heroin, but its trajectory differs from other countries in the region that have been affected by fentanyl.

This is not an exhaustive list: Other countries have active illicit fentanyl markets. For instance, Lithuania reported a recent increase in trafficking cases and drug seizures linked to carfentanil, which also has been reported by toxicology analyses there (EMCDDA, 2018e). Fentanyl use has been noted in Australia, although the extent to which it is illicitly manufactured or the result of diverted pharmaceutical products remains unclear (Australian Institute of Health and Welfare, 2018).[1]

---

[1]   Because of scope limitations, we focused on countries where illicitly manufactured fentanyl has established a notable presence as a dominant opioid (with Sweden as a unique case and Finland as a very unique comparator). To our knowledge, there is no country in Western

There are other examples of illicit fentanyl use in the past, albeit often limited in duration or geographic extent. The EMCDDA has noted fentanyl use in Bavaria, as well as brief outbreaks in the early 2010s in Bulgaria and Slovakia (Mounteney, Evans-Brown, and Giraudon, 2012). Since 2012, 23 European Union member states have reported fentanyl in their national drug markets (Evans-Brown, Gallegos, and Christie, 2018). Notwithstanding these other cases, our sample includes the closest comparator to the United States (i.e., Canada), as well as several geographically clustered European countries, which demonstrate considerable diversity in the penetration and staying power of fentanyl markets within a confined region (see Figure 4.1). This diversity is a caution against overconfidence that fentanyl's arrival inevitably leads to one outcome or another and is one reason why we discuss multiple possible future scenarios in Chapter Five.

Figure 4.1
Selected Focus Countries

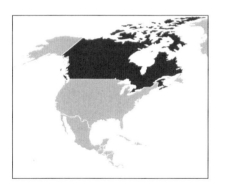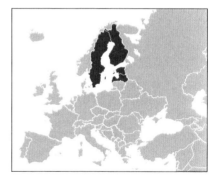

Europe that has seen fentanyl penetrate as much and heroin lose ground to a comparable extent.

Country Profiles

Estonia
Historical Overview and Market Characteristics

Fentanyl emerged in Estonia in the aftermath of the 2001 Taliban poppy ban, which reduced the availability of heroin in Europe (Ojanperä et al., 2008).[2] Since 2002, fentanyl and its analogs have dominated illicit opioid markets in Estonia, with 3-methylfentanyl (3MF) appearing in 2003 and remaining one of the two main analogs available (Tuusov et al., 2013). Initially, fentanyl was marketed as heroin, although, according to drug policy professionals either involved in or familiar with research involving people who use drugs (PWUD) in Estonia, users eventually learned that this was a novel substance rather than potent heroin. Fentanyl and its analogs have largely displaced heroin, making the country the only known mature synthetic opioid market in the world.[3] This makes Estonia a particularly important case to study.

Interviewees commenting on the situation in Estonia and existing literature suggest that the fentanyl available in Estonia in the 2000s was smuggled in from Russia in highly pure forms (Ojanperä et al., 2008; Tuusov et al., 2013) and that distribution was controlled by Russian-speaking organized crime groups in Estonia. However, it remains unclear whether the fentanyl was produced in Russia or if Russia was only a transit country. Some literature, as well as law enforcement and public health interviewees, note the existence of fentanyl production in the post-Soviet space (Europol, 2007), while other literature and experts suggest that China was the country of origin even for these

---

[2]   Although fentanyl did not achieve its dominance until 2002, one interviewee suggested that it had begun to be available in the late 1990s. However, this is not supported by data from the Estonian Forensic Service Centre, which indicate the first seizures of fentanyl in 2001 and 2002. Later in this chapter, we discuss additional factors that potentially played a significant role in the emergence of fentanyl in Estonia and other countries. We also note the debate surrounding the overall consequences of the Taliban poppy ban (Paoli, Greenfield, and Reuter, 2009).

[3]   According to one interviewee working in law enforcement, the little remaining use of heroin in Estonia is concentrated among the country's Roma population.

early shipments (Denissov, 2014).[4] With notable exceptions, there has been little domestic production of fentanyl, although local distributors have been responsible for cutting and packaging the drug. When fentanyl was smuggled from Russia in a liquid form, Estonia-based distributors also were responsible for converting it to powder.

In 2015, new fentanyl analogs began to appear, leading to a proliferation of synthetic opioids (see Figure 4.2). The analogs represent an addition to, rather than a substitute for, traditional fentanyl and 3MF, which still accounted for most new treatment entrants in 2016 (EMCDDA, 2018a). It is generally believed that these new analogs are shipped from China via mail, either directly to Estonia or via third

Figure 4.2
Counts of Fentanyl and Fentanyl Analog Seizures in Estonia, 2009–2018

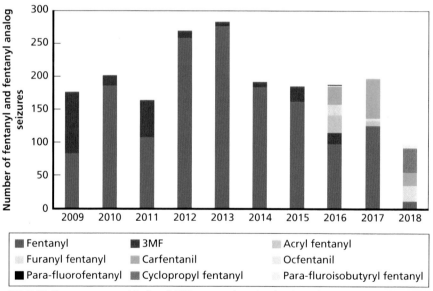

SOURCE: Data were provided to RAND researchers by the Estonian Forensic Service Centre.

---

[4]   However, this appears to be a minority view and there is little evidence from other sources of Chinese fentanyl production this early.

countries (EMCDDA, 2018a).[5] There is no meaningful differentiation between the traditional fentanyl and analog markets; both serve the same population, both are marketed the same way, and both of their distribution systems are managed by the same organized crime groups. The advent of internet sales and international shipping has opened up the possibility of users buying synthetic opioids directly from producers; however, according to one law enforcement and one drug policy professional, this is very rare.[6]

User Population, Preferences, and Harms

People who use illicit fentanyl in Estonia are largely long-term opioid users, are predominantly located in the north and northeast of the country, and belong to the Russian-speaking population (EMCDDA, 2018a; Mounteney, Evans-Brown, and Giraudon, 2012). The origins of the large injecting population in Estonia date to the dissolution of the Soviet Union and the ensuing social, economic, and political transformation. As pointed out by public health and drug policy interviewees, the number of injection drug users peaked at approximately 20,000 in the late 1990s (shortly *before* the arrival of fentanyl) and has been in decline since then.

Estimates in the 2000s showed a decrease from nearly 16,000 people who inject drugs (PWID) in 2005 to slightly more than 5,000 in 2009 (Uusküla et al., 2013). A subsequent estimate (based on expert opinion rather than on previously used methods) published in 2014 put the number of PWID at 9,000, of whom 6,000 were thought to be opioid injectors (Raben et al., 2014).[7] Most recently, the 2019 EMCDDA country drug report noted that there were an estimated 8,600 PWID ages 15 to 44 in Estonia in 2015, the majority of whom

---

[5]   The extent to which Russia has continued to supply traditional fentanyl in the face of the rise in international shipping from China is not clear.

[6]   Estonia is a very digitally connected country, so the lack of direct online purchases by users even in that mature market is worth noting. It could be attributable to the fact that users are a marginalized population.

[7]   Caution is required in interpreting the data because the earlier estimate by Uuskula et al. (2013) implies a decline of two-thirds over four years. Estonia does not produce annual estimates of the number of heavy drug users for the EMCDDA.

were noted as using opioids (EMCDDA, 2019a). The decline in the user population in Estonia was confirmed by all five interviewees who commented on the issue, all of whom also noted that there are relatively few new opioid users in the country and that the existing user population is aging.

The introduction of fentanyl in the early 2000s led to a sudden increase in drug-related deaths in Estonia, with deaths more than doubling between 2001 and 2002 (see Figure 4.3). Drug-related deaths peaked at 170 in 2012, at which point Estonia had one of the highest overdose death rates in the world.[8] The number of deaths decreased somewhat after the 2012 peak, only to increase again in 2016 and 2017, which appears to coincide with the emergence of new fentanyl analogs.

If the prevalence of use decreased by roughly 50 percent between the mid 2000s and the mid 2010s, then the decline in deaths was less

Figure 4.3
Drug-Related Death Rate in Estonia per 100,000 People, 2000–2018

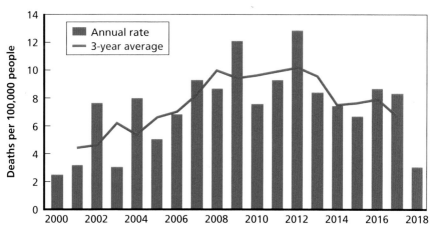

SOURCE: Data on deaths are from the Estonian Cause of Death Registry, 2019. Data on population are from Statistics Estonia, 2019.
NOTE: 2002 was the first full year with the presence of fentanyl noted; 2016 was the first full year with the presence of analogs other than 3MF noted.

---

[8]   The peak death rate in Estonia in 2012 (12.85 per 100,000 people; see Figure 4.3) was somewhat lower than the current opioid death rate in the United States (14.9 per 100,000 people, according to 2017 data).

than proportional. That is, deaths per 1,000 users might have increased even as the total number of deaths edged downward.

That fentanyl increased deaths without increasing prevalence could be an important observation with implications for North America. Conceivably, the very fact that fentanyl is so deadly might dissuade some from initiating opioid use.

As discussed earlier, Estonian users learned that fentanyl and its analogs had completely replaced heroin.[9] So now, users expect to obtain synthetic opioids when purchasing drugs from the street, but they do not know which analog might be present. This can increase risks when a new analog with different potency or effects is introduced into the market. This appears to be borne out in the mortality data, which spiked following the 2003 introduction of 3MF, which is more potent than fentanyl, as well as when newer analogs appeared in 2015 and 2016.

Multiple informants (two drug policy professionals and one law enforcement interviewee) pointed out that Estonian users now expect to buy fentanyl (or, more recently, an analog) and have become accustomed to it. Correspondingly, tolerance in users and simple familiarity might make a return to heroin unlikely. That said, one drug policy professional suggested that, based on qualitative work with the user population, older users miss the predictability of the old heroin supply. Users' preference for fentanyl, coupled with the greater ease with which the drug can be produced and trafficked, was highlighted by interviewees as the primary reason why heroin has not returned to Estonia. A few interviewees (law enforcement and drug policy professionals) pointed out that fentanyl is effectively cheaper than heroin. Although the nominal price for fentanyl remains the same as for heroin (€10 per dose of 0.015–0.03 g of a mixture containing fentanyl), higher potency makes fentanyl more affordable because many users split the purchase

---

[9]   In the context of user learning, two policy professionals noted efforts to build and maintain channels of communication and feedback loops among the user population, social workers, health services, and the police to collect information from users on what is available on the street and communicate information to users as well (e.g., changes in the market, emergence of new analogs, risk-mitigation strategies).

into smaller doses.[10] According to the samples analyzed by the Estonian Forensic Science Institute, in 2016, the most common purity of fentanyl in Estonia was 2.9 percent and it ranged from 0.94 percent to 12 percent.[11]

Current Situation

As of early 2019, the fentanyl market in Estonia was undergoing a period of instability. In 2017, Estonian law enforcement managed to disrupt fentanyl distribution networks by arresting most of the high-level drug traffickers in the country (Kund, 2017). These operations resulted in record-high seizures (shown in Table 4.1) and shut down a

Table 4.1
Total Volume of Fentanyl and Fentanyl Analog Seizures in Estonia, 2014–2018

Substance (g)	2014	2015	2016	2017	2018[a]
Fentanyl	735	940	314	9,792	91
3MF	1	52	99	0	0
Acryl fentanyl	0	0	130	3	0
Furanyl fentanyl	0	0	82	260	93
Carfentanil	0	0	71	165	33
Ocfentanil	0	0	1	0	0
Para-fluorofentanyl	0	0	1	0	0
Cyclopropyl fentanyl	0	0	0	0	274
Para-fluoroisobutyryl fentanyl	0	0	< 1	0	82
Total	736	992	698	10,220	572

SOURCE: Data were provided to RAND researchers by the Estonian Forensic Science Institute.
NOTE: Denotes total volume of seizures not adjusted for purity.
[a] January–October only.

---

[10] Of course, if the switch to fentanyl was accompanied by more frequent use, this would negate some of the savings.

[11] Unlike with cocaine or heroin, low purity values should not necessarily be understood as an indicator of fentanyl's poor quality. Given fentanyl's very high potency, large volumes of filler are needed to make the dose sizable enough to be handled by end users. The purity information presented here is from data provided to the authors.

domestic fentanyl laboratory. This was a one-off discovery, as no other instances of domestic production of fentanyl have been reported.

As a result, for several months, fentanyl was scarce (in the estimate of one interviewee, this period lasted for about four to six months). Some users reportedly complained about difficulties accessing fentanyl and travelled to Riga, Latvia, to obtain it. Correspondingly, the number of drug-related deaths has decreased significantly, from 110 in 2017 to 40 in 2018.

Since then, the supply has been partially restored. Prices (not adjusted for purity) are still higher than they were before the disruption and are currently reported to be about €20–25 per dose. Somewhat counterintuitively, the purity of fentanyl products analyzed by the Estonian Forensic Science Institute increased: The most common purity in 2017 was 13 percent.[12] In a new development, multidose packages have become commonly available, effectively offering users volume discounts. The wholesale price of fentanyl is currently reported to be €60–120 per gram.[13]

Finland
Historical Overview and Market Characteristics
The opioid market in Finland has followed a unique path. In the 1990s, it was dominated by heroin coming from Afghanistan via Estonia or Russia (Finnish National Focal Point, 2004). Similar to the 2001 disruption in Estonia, the market in Finland was disrupted in the same year, as is clear by notable decreases in heroin seizures and purity (Finnish National Focal Point, 2004). However, in Estonia, heroin was replaced by fentanyl; in Finland, heroin was replaced by buprenorphine, which is used to treat pain but can be dispensed for the treatment of OUD. Heroin became rare to the point that the

---

[12] Available data on purity do not include data on size. Although we do not have further data to corroborate, one possible explanation would be an increasing shift to online purchases of mass-produced Chinese product.

[13] It is somewhat difficult to reconcile wholesale and retail indicators because data on purity in the wholesale market are not available. Assuming that the wholesale purity exceeds that at the retail level implies a substantial markup at the retail level. The data in this paragraph were provided to the authors.

EMCDDA's 2005 country report noted that buprenorphine was the main drug used by four out of five opioid users in the country (Finnish National Focal Point, 2006).[14] The switch appears to have been permanent. Buprenorphine remains the most commonly used illicit opioid, and all interviewees commenting on Finland stressed that heroin continues to be rare.[15] This also has been confirmed in recent wastewater analyses covering nearly half of the Finnish population (Gunnar and Kankaanpää, 2018; Kankaanpää et al., 2016).

The buprenorphine used in Finland is a pharmaceutical-grade monoformulation, diverted from other countries, including France and the Baltic countries, particularly Lithuania (Gunnar et al., 2018; Finnish National Focal Point, 2006).[16] There is no or very little diversion of buprenorphine from the domestic health care system, perhaps because the main medication used in treatment in Finland is buprenorphine in combination with naloxone (which accounts for 62 percent of all prescriptions), followed by methadone (32 percent). Mono-buprenorphine (which is used in less than 2 percent of cases) is primarily disbursed to pregnant women and individuals with an allergy to naloxone (Partanen et al., 2017).

Estonian and Finnish organized crime groups have been linked to buprenorphine trafficking, although the role of user-led networks and the personal importation of buprenorphine from France also has been noted, particularly in the early 2000s (Hermanson and Järvinen, 2003).[17] Illicit buprenorphine is mainly injected after being crushed.

The wholesale price in 2017 was €22,000 for 1,000 tablets. The retail price was reported to be €50 per tablet, although one law enforcement and one drug policy interviewee pointed out some regional varia-

---

[14] One noteworthy exception was a large seizure of more than 50 kg of heroin on the Russo-Finnish border, with a final destination of Sweden (Finnish National Focal Point, 2006).

[15] Leskinen (2018) notes attempts by African organized crime groups to supply heroin to Finland.

[16] Mono-formulation buprenorphine does not contain naloxone, which is common in formulations offered in the United States under the trade name Suboxone.

[17] Estonian groups are primarily responsible for smuggling into the country, and Finnish groups are responsible for domestic distribution (Leskinen, 2018).

tion in price levels, with higher prices in northern Finland (which is also reported by Leskinen, 2018). These are similar to prices recorded in 2004, which were €50–80 per buprenorphine tablet (Finnish National Focal Point, 2006).[18] According to an interviewed drug policy professional, one tablet can provide multiple (about four, depending on tolerance) doses for injection, making the price roughly €10 per injection.[19] This is comparable to the price per dose in Estonia before the recent market disruptions there.

All interviewees commenting on Finland (representing both public health and law enforcement) noted that fentanyl and its analogs have not been a major issue in Finland, although they remain a concern because of their appearance in neighboring countries. That said, some limited fentanyl presence in Finland has been reported in the past, particularly in the early 2010s. The 2012 EMCDDA Trendspotter survey mentioned localized use of fentanyl centered on the city of Turku (Mounteney, Evans-Brown, and Giraudon, 2012). Forssell and Nurmi (2014) notes that 1 percent of drug service clients in 2013 reported using fentanyl, and furanyl fentanyl and carfentanil were detected in a very small number of postmortem cases. In 2017, there were only a "few sporadic findings" of novel synthetic opioids in Finland (Krikku and Ronka, 2018, p. 3).

User Population, Preferences, and Harms

There were 13,000 to 15,000 high-risk opioid users in Finland in 2012, or approximately four per 1,000 adult population (Ollgren et al., 2014).[20] This is notably higher than previous estimates of 1,500 to 3,300 in 1997 and 4,200 to 5,900 in 2002 (Finnish National Focal

---

[18] This similarity applies to recorded heroin prices (unadjusted for purity) as well: €150 per gram in 2017 and €120–200 per gram in 2004.

[19] This is also broadly in line with findings by Alho et al. (2007). Finnish injection users of buprenorphine involved in the study ($n = 176$ questionnaires) reported consuming, on average, 7 mg of buprenorphine per day, with the majority of respondents reporting using twice (26.1 percent) or 3–4 times (41.6 percent) per day. This equals an injection dose of about 2 mg, or one-quarter of an 8-mg tablet.

[20] A similar estimate is replicated in the most recent EMCDDA country reports (EMCDDA, 2018c; EMCDDA, 2019b).

Point, 2006). However, these estimates are not directly comparable because of differences in methods and improvements in recording (Varjonen, 2015). Still, other sources suggest that there has been an increase in the number of high-risk opioid users. An updated estimate is due to be published in 2019; according to interviewed public health professionals, there is little evidence of a substantial increase in the opioid user population from the 2012 data.

In 2017, Finland had 200 drug-related deaths, with the majority involving buprenorphine, typically in combination with other drugs (EMCDDA, 2019b). As Figure 4.4 shows, the number of deaths

Figure 4.4
Drug-Related Death Rate in Finland per 100,000 People, 2000–2017

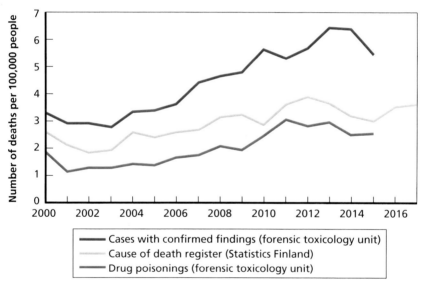

SOURCE: EMCDDA, 2019b; Krikku and Ronka, 2018; population data are from Statistics Finland, 2019.
NOTE: The top line represents all cases in which the presence of a drug was identified in postmortems, irrespective of whether it was the direct (or major indirect) cause of death. The middle line shows cases from the general mortality register in which the drug was the cause of death (either direct or indirect) and includes both intentional and unintentional poisonings and mental health episodes attributable to drug use. This is the metric used by the EMCDDA. The bottom line shows all instances of drug poisonings confirmed by the forensic toxicology unit. It excludes cases without known signs or history of drug use.

approximately doubled between the early 2000s and 2012, broadly corresponding to the estimated growth in the user population over the same period.

In line with the market trends described earlier, the number of heroin-related deaths plummeted after 2002, dropping to "almost nil" by 2007 (Varjonen, 2015, p. 92). In 2015, heroin appeared in just five postmortems (Krikku and Ronka, 2018). Also in line with the trends described earlier, the number of fentanyl-related deaths increased in the early 2010s (Simonsen et al., 2015) but continues to be very small. In 2010, there were 16 fentanyl-related deaths in Finland (Vuori et al., 2012), and in 2015, fentanyl was confirmed in eight fatal poisonings (Krikku and Ronka, 2018).

Current Situation

According to all interviewees (both public health and law enforcement professionals) commenting on the situation in Finland, there have been no major changes in the Finnish drug market recently, an assessment with which the latest EMCDDA country report concurs (EMCDDA, 2019b). The emergence of novel psychoactive substances and online drug sales have been noted but have yet to have a major impact (Krikku and Ronka, 2018).[21]

Sweden
Historical Overview and Market Characteristics

Fentanyl made its first short-lived appearance in Sweden in the mid-1990s when—sold as heroin—it resulted in nine deaths (Kronstrand et al., 1997). It reappeared briefly in the early 2000s, sold either alone or mixed with heroin and marketed as either heroin or "China White," before disappearing by 2004. According to a law enforcement interviewee, the source in both instances is thought to have been the same as that supplying Estonia (i.e., Russia or the larger post-Soviet space).

In 2006, diverted fentanyl patches appeared on the Swedish illicit market and have stayed ever since, although their market share has

---

[21] Stimulants have been the most prevalent type of new psychoactive substance detected in Finland, with relatively few cases of novel synthetic opioids, although carfentanil has been noted as a "rising threat" (Leskinen, 2018).

remained relatively limited. There has been very little evidence of fentanyl patch smuggling into Sweden, suggesting that patches have been diverted from the local health care system.

Fentanyl analogs arrived around January 2014, sold online by Swedish vendors and distributed directly to customers via Swedish Post.[22] China is generally thought to be the source of these analogs, which are shipped by mail to vendors in Sweden (although not necessarily directly, frequently a third European Union transit country is involved). After experimentation with various formulations, such as blotter paper and powder, nasal sprays emerged as a dominant form, followed by tablets (although to a much lesser extent). Both nasal sprays and tablets were explicitly marketed as fentanyl analogs, although it is possible that the analog in the delivered product did not match the original description. Importantly, this analog market was entirely separate from the street-based heroin market, and there is little evidence of the online analog market mixing with the heroin in street markets (Polisen, 2018). Thus. three important and distinct opioid markets had established themselves in Sweden by 2014 (see Table 4.2).

There also was some limited distribution of counterfeit prescription tablets containing fentanyl between 2015 and 2018. These were predominantly fake oxycodone or tramadol tablets, along with some counterfeit Xanax tablets. In addition, an illicit market of pharmaceutical-grade prescription opioids has been noted by Swedish

Table 4.2
Principal Heroin and Fentanyl Markets in Sweden, 2014–2017

Product	Main Formulation	Most Common Source	Distribution
Heroin	Powder	Afghanistan or Pakistan	On the street
Fentanyl	Patch	Swedish health care system	On the street and online
Fentanyl analogs	Nasal spray	China, by mail	Online

SOURCE: Polisen, 2018.

---

[22] Sales of AH-7921, a novel synthetic opioid, preceded fentanyl analogs and started in Sweden in 2012. AH-7921 was offered by online vendors selling other new psychoactive substances, such as synthetic cannabinoids.

law enforcement interviewees. This market is dominated by tramadol, which is smuggled into Sweden.

User Population, Preferences, and Harms

Sweden does not submit official annual estimates of the prevalence of problem opioid use to the EMCDDA, but the EMCDDA's 2017 Swedish country report cited a 2011 study, which estimated that there were approximately 8,000 PWID in the country, most of them using either opioids or stimulants (EMCDDA, 2017). An estimate based on expert opinion cited in 2017 by the Swedish Police put the population of heroin users at 5,000.[23] In addition, the Intelligence Division of its National Operations Department estimated that there were approximately 1,000 fentanyl analog users in Sweden (Polisen, 2018).

The introduction of fentanyl analogs in 2014 was followed by a notable increase in drug-related deaths (Figure 4.5), but this merely continued (and accentuated) a long-term trend driven by increases in deaths involving pharmaceutical opioids (Leifman, 2016a).[24] As in North America, that trend occurred against the backdrop of notable increases in prescription rates for pharmaceutical opioids (analgesics as well as medications to treat opioid-use disorder) in Sweden.[25]

The use of fentanyl and fentanyl analogs was associated with a much higher risk of death than that for the use of heroin alone. Despite

---

[23] This could be an underestimate. If Sweden had only 5,000 heroin users, the observed number of heroin deaths would imply an unusually high fatality rate compared with that of most other European nations, and the reported number of medication therapy clients (more than 4,000 in 2016; EMCDDA, 2018f) would imply a coverage rate higher than that of most other European nations.

[24] The magnitude of the increase in drug-related deaths might have been overestimated by two unrelated changes in data recording practices in the first half of the 2010s. The first revolved around coding practices for causes of death listed on death certificates and increased inclusion of various causes in the drug-related deaths statistics. Notable examples include tramadol (excluded until 2012) and dextropropoxyphene (which was not included until its removal from the Swedish market in the early 2010s). The second change was improvements to toxicological examinations consisting of more-systematic testing as well as improved analytical equipment able to detect smaller concentrations of substances (Leifman, 2016b).

[25] Between 2006 and 2014, prescription rates increased for buprenorphine, methadone, morphine, and fentanyl, as well as for oxycodone (Fugelstad, 2015).

Figure 4.5
Drug-Related Death Rate in Sweden per 100,000 People, 2004–2017

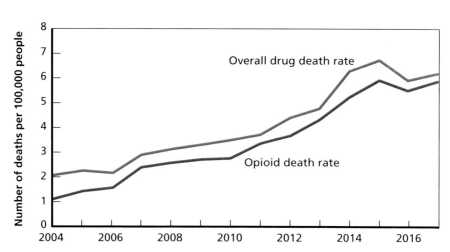

SOURCES: EMCDDA, 2017; EMCDDA, 2018f; EMCDDA, 2019f; Leifman, 2016a;
Statistics Sweden, 2019.
NOTES: The figure presents drug-related and opioid-involved deaths based on the
Swedish official register of causes of death (GMR) as defined by the EMCDDA. It
includes cases in which the drug was assessed as the underlying cause of death,
irrespective of whether the case was forensically investigated or whether the drug
toxicology is known.

the estimated population of heroin users being five times larger than
the estimated number of fentanyl users (5,000 versus 1,000), the
number of heroin-related deaths in 2017 (108 deaths) was lower than
deaths attributed to fentanyl and related substances (101 from analogs,
30 from patches).[26] The near elimination of fentanyl deaths in 2018
looks like a major public health success and, as discussed later, it might
stem from enforcement efforts against Sweden's major importers and
distributors.

Figure 4.6 captures these trends by showing the number of deaths
in Sweden involving heroin, fentanyl, or fentanyl analogs since 2014.

---

[26] These numbers are based on the toxreg database, which comments on the presence of the
drug irrespective of any causality. For that reason, there could be some overlap in the fentanyl
and heroin numbers presented here, although little mixing between the heroin and fentanyl
markets has been reported in Sweden.

Figure 4.6
Heroin and Fentanyl and Fentanyl Analogs in Drug Deaths in Sweden, 2014–2018

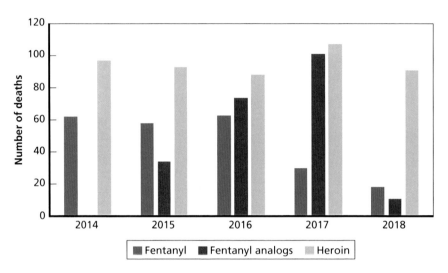

SOURCE: National Board of Forensic Medicine, 2019.
NOTE: The database of forensic toxicologies shows whether a given drug was detected in the death examination (either alone or in combination). It does not comment on the cause of death. A small number of 2018 cases remain incomplete.

Heroin deaths remained relatively stable, while analogs rose rapidly from 2015 to 2017.

As discussed earlier, there were very few links between the online fentanyl analog market and the street heroin market. Although the heroin market primarily served long-term users, according to law enforcement interviewees familiar with the situation, the online fentanyl analog marketplace attracted a mix of users, some without prior experience with opioids and more with such experience. Some were looking to manage pain after their licit analgesic prescriptions were discontinued; this group might have had reservations about injecting, which made the nasal spray formulation attractive (and, sometimes, legal). For others with a history of OUD, including those engaging with medication treatment programs, fentanyl analogs represented an alternative that might not have been controlled by legislation and thus was not likely to be detected during routine urinalysis.[27] Relatedly, multiple law enforcement interviewees noted that the supply of individual analogs appeared to respond to changes in the Swedish regulatory regime, with suppliers aiming to stay one step ahead of the law by introducing new types of analogs. (Figure 4.7 illustrates the variety of fentanyl and fentanyl analogs seized in Sweden in 2017). Furthermore, for opioid users in rural places and small towns, the online analog marketplace created availability where there were no street-level heroin markets. According to law enforcement interviewees, the fentanyl patch market, which preceded the analog market, straddled the boundary between the analog and heroin markets, attracting users from both of these markets.

Figure 4.7
Fentanyl and Its Analogs Seized in Sweden, 2017

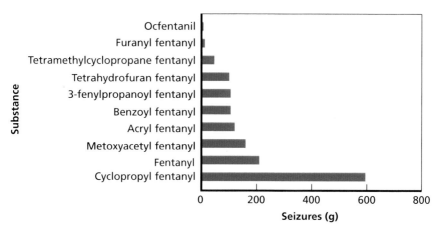

SOURCE: Data were provided directly to RAND researchers by Swedish Customs.
NOTES: Denotes total volume of seizures not adjusted for purity. Numbers are in volume by grams.

---

[27] An important context for this observation is the fact that use, in addition to possession, is a criminal offense in Sweden (EMCDDA, 2018d).

Current Situation

Since early 2018, there have been no reports of fentanyl analogs available on the Swedish market. At the end of 2017 and in early 2018, Swedish authorities arrested and brought cases against the three biggest vendors of fentanyl analogs in the country. Besides arrests and prosecution for the distribution of controlled substances, one vendor selling uncontrolled analogs was convicted of involuntary manslaughter related to analog overdoses (an appeal was pending as of early 2019). According to multiple law enforcement interviewees, this demonstrated to Swedish vendors that they were not immune from legal repercussions even if their products did not contain any controlled substances. Subsequently, the remaining vendors stopped selling and nobody has taken their place.

The discontinuation of online analog sales has translated into a notable decrease in drug-related deaths in Sweden from 2017 to 2018. As of the writing of this analysis, the last fentanyl-related death in Sweden occurred in August 2018. One interviewee pointed out that this was a dramatic decrease since late 2017, when fentanyl deaths averaged approximately one every day.

Latvia
Historical Overview and Market Characteristics

Fentanyl analogs were first detected on the Latvian market in 2012 with the identification of carfentanil in the national drug supply. However, availability remained very limited until 2015, when carfentanil began to claim an increasing share of the illegal market. Carfentanil dominated until 2017, when a large number of analogs appeared and diversified the market supply (there has never been a seizure of the original fentanyl compound in the country; see Figure 4.8). Most recently, cyclopropyl fentanyl has become a commonly available analog, as seen in the increase of seizures involving this substance in 2017 and 2018.

China is generally considered to be the source of fentanyl analogs in Latvia (EMCDDA, 2018d).[28] Some analogs might be mailed

---

[28] This is also in line with testimonies by all interviewees commenting on the situation in Latvia. One drug policy professional shared that, according to the Latvian police, it is pos-

Figure 4.8
Number of Fentanyl Seizures in Latvia, 2012–2018

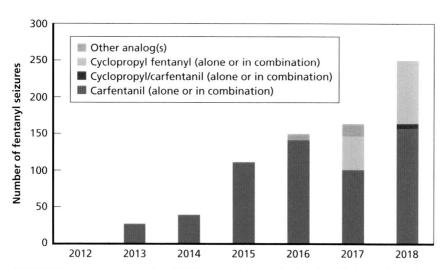

SOURCE: Data were provided to RAND researchers by the Latvian Ministry of Interior.

directly to Latvia; however, a law enforcement interviewee noted that most are transshipped by land from other European Union countries, with Latvian-based dealers responsible for the cutting of the drugs and the distribution to retail markets.[29] According to one interviewed drug policy and one law enforcement professional, there is little evidence of users buying products directly from Chinese suppliers. There is no known domestic production of fentanyl and its analogs, and only limited diversion of fentanyl patches from the domestic health care system. One patch is reported to cost €20.[30]

---

sible to observe changes in the Latvian market in terms of supplied substances following regulatory changes in China.

[29] This is perhaps not surprising, as drugs flow in trade routes. The Sino-Latvian trade might be very small, so fentanyls travel in the larger flows to other European Union countries and then in the relatively smaller flows to Latvia.

[30] This information was provided to the RAND team. The number of doses available from one patch depends on the formulation. According to an Australian peer education document on injecting fentanyl, a 12.5-mcg-per-hour patch (the lowest dose available on the market)

Synthetic opioids have largely replaced heroin, which is now available only to a limited extent and is frequently mixed with carfentanil or other analogs. According to one drug policy professional we interviewed, the mixing of heroin and fentanyl analogs was quite common from 2015 to 2017 but has become less common, perhaps reflecting the decrease in heroin's market share. Historically, there was no difference in how fentanyl analogs were marketed; the distribution networks were the same for heroin and fentanyl analogs. However, according to an interviewed drug policy professional and one law enforcement interviewee, and as documented in the literature, users have realized the presence of a new substance and have started referring to fentanyl analogs by a new street name.[31] Dealers have been reported to warn users that their product is stronger than traditional heroin and instances of carfentanil sold as carfentanil also have been reported (Gribova, 2018). As reported by a drug policy interviewee, when unadjusted for purity, synthetic opioids (€10–15 per dose) are currently reported to be cheaper than heroin (€30 per dose), although the historical nominal price for a heroin dose used to be similar to the current price for a fentanyl analog dose.[32] The price per dose in Latvia is very similar to that reported in Estonia before the recent law enforcement–led disruption of the Estonian market, although data are not available to compare the purity of street-sold fentanyls.

Alongside fentanyl analogs, there is a robust market for illicit opioid treatment medications (e.g., methadone and buprenorphine). According to an interviewed drug policy professional and one law enforcement interviewee, the main sources for illicit opioid treatment medications appear to be other European countries, although, in 2017, Latvian authorities identified two illicit methadone laboratories in the country. One drug policy interviewee admitted the possibility that buprenorphine could be diverted from Latvian medication treatment

---

contains approximately 2.1 mg of fentanyl. That broadly corresponds to one dose sold in Estonia or British Columbia (Australian Injecting and Illicit Drug Users League, 2013).

[31] This information was provided to the RAND team.

[32] For comparison, the retail price of heroin in 2017 reported by the police was €60–150 per gram (unadjusted for purity; Gribova, 2018).

programs but added that there has not been much evidence of this. Methadone has been reported as occasionally mixed with heroin and fentanyl analogs.

According to one interviewee, nonprescribed use of prescription opioids has not been a major issue, although the EMCDDA 2018 country report (EMCDDA, 2018d) mentioned tramadol as another substance replacing heroin and a small number of tramadol and carfentanil seizures have been reported.

User Population, Preferences, and Harms

The fentanyl analog user population in Latvia is similar to that in Estonia, consisting primarily of low-income individuals with severe OUD, often without a fixed residence. According to an EMCDDA estimate, there were slightly more than 7,000 high-risk opioid users in Latvia, corresponding to a rate of 5.6 per 1,000 adults (EMCDDA, 2019c). The user population is concentrated in Riga, with synthetic opioid use reported in other cities as well, depending on the existence of regional distribution networks. According to the 2018 country report, until 2016, opioid use in Latvia had been declining, although the estimate for 2017 is slightly higher than that for 2016 (EMCDDA, 2018d; EMCDDA, 2019c). This is consistent with the testimonies of interviewees who note that, as in Estonia, there are relatively few new opioid users and the overall user population has been aging. As in Estonia, fentanyl analogs are injected, and diverted fentanyl patches tend to be boiled up to a liquid form and then subsequently injected.

The introduction of carfentanil to Latvia in 2012 led to an increase in the number of drug-related deaths, albeit from a low base. In 2013 and 2014, the number of deaths decreased, only to increase in 2015 following a large-scale spread of carfentanil (see Figure 4.9). However, the number of drug-related deaths after 2015 was still lower than that recorded in the late 2000s. In fact, the Latvian drug-related death rate in 2017 was lower than the European average.

According to a law enforcement interviewee citing results of interviews with fentanyl analog users in Latvia, some actually prefer fentanyl analogs, while others prefer heroin and use new synthetic opioids primarily for availability reasons. The interviewee added that older

Figure 4.9
Drug-Related Death Rate in Latvia per 100,000 People, 2006–2017

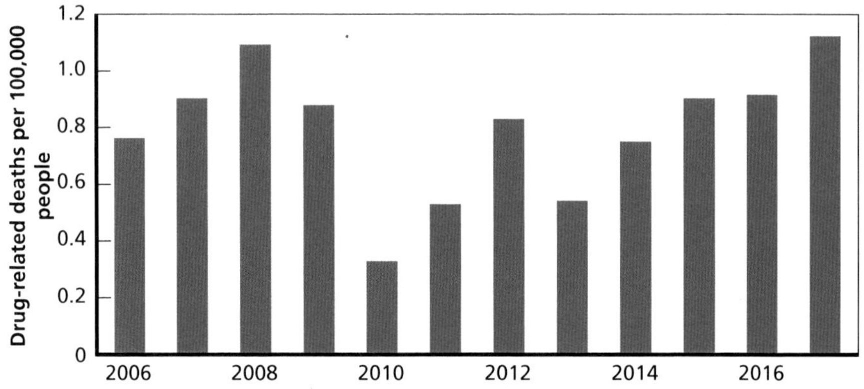

SOURCES: EMCDDA, 2018d; EMCDDA, 2019c; Central Statistical Bureau of Latvia, 2019.
NOTES: Because of the comparatively low death rate and Latvia's relatively small population, the absolute number of drug-related deaths in Latvia is by far the smallest of all countries presented in this analysis. In 2008, the year of the highest number of deaths, there were 24 deaths.

users were more likely to prefer heroin while the younger generation was more open to new synthetic opioids as a drug of choice.

Current Situation

The current situation in Latvia reflects a continuation of the trends described earlier. Fentanyl analogs continue to grow at the expense of heroin, and the number of analogs appears to be increasing. Unlike in Estonia, there has been no evidence of any disruption to the national fentanyl analog market; in fact, as multiple interviewees pointed out, fentanyl analogs from Latvia have recently been used to supplement the reduced supply in Estonia.

Canada
Historical Overview and Market Characteristics

According to an interviewed drug policy professional, illicitly manufactured fentanyl was first detected in British Columbia in 2012, and in 2013, the Canadian Community Epidemiology Network on Drug

Use (CCENDU) warned of the emergence of fentanyl and fentanyl analogs, initially offered as counterfeit oxycodone tablets (CCENDU, 2013; CCENDU, 2014). Several interviewees added that, as in the United States, this demand for diverted pharmaceuticals came amid growing restrictions on prescribing as well as the introduction of tamper-proof oxycodone formulation on the Canadian market.

Over time, counterfeit pills appear to have diminished, and powder is now the main formulation available on the Canadian market. As multiple interviewees (representing law enforcement, drug policy, and public health professionals) reported, fentanyl is marketed as "down," a term historically used for heroin, which has taken on the meaning of any opioid. Therefore, there appears to be no difference in how heroin and fentanyl are marketed. Correspondingly, the reported price for a dose of heroin and fentanyl (half a tenth of a gram, or a "half point" of an opioid-containing mixture) in Vancouver is identical at C$10. According to one law enforcement interviewee commenting on the situation in British Columbia, the fentanyl content of this mixture is approximately 2 percent. This makes the purity-adjusted price of fentanyl in British Columbia broadly in line with that reported in Estonia.[33]

Fentanyl and its analogs have been displacing heroin in some drug markets. According to one interviewee's estimate, currently, the market in British Columbia is approximately 80 percent fentanyl and/or analogs only, 10 percent fentanyl and/or analogs mixed with heroin, and 10 percent heroin only. Another interviewee from British Columbia agreed that heroin-only samples or certificates of death were exceedingly rare. The growth of fentanyls also is reflected in samples submitted to the Canadian Drug Analysis Service, although not to the same extent (see Figure 4.10).[34]

---

[33] In British Columbia, the price of C$10 for 0.05 g of a mixture containing 2 percent fentanyl corresponds to a price of C$10 for 1 mg of pure fentanyl. In Estonia, the price of €10 for 0.015–0.03 g of a mixture containing 2.9 percent fentanyl (modal value reported in 2016) corresponds to a price of €10 for slightly less than 1 mg of pure fentanyl.

[34] These data cannot be understood as representative of all seizures in Canada. The Drug Analysis Service analyzes samples provided by Canadian law enforcement agencies; no information is available on seizures that are not submitted to the Drug Analysis Service.

Figure 4.10
Opioids Submitted for Analysis to the Canadian Drug Analysis Service in the Three Most Affected Provinces, 2016–2019

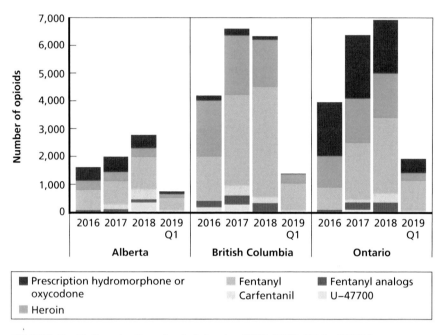

SOURCE: Health Canada, Drug Analysis Service (2017, 2018, 2019a, 2019b).

It is not clear whether these counts are all distinct cases or whether a sample could appear in multiple categories if it contained multiple chemicals. However, if one adds the number of mentions for fentanyl and its analogs and divides them by the totals, in all three provinces, the fentanyls' share of mentions grew by about 20 percentage points from 2016 to early 2018, from about 50 percent to 70 percent in Alberta and British Columbia and from 22 percent to 42 percent in Ontario, where hydromorphone and oxycodone are common.

All interviewees commenting on Canada (representing all stakeholder groups) noted that China is the source of illicitly manufactured fentanyl. Typically, the product is shipped in powder form to organized crime groups in Canada, which manage its distribution. The pressing of counterfeit tablets takes place in Canada.[35] Every interviewee confirmed that there is no meaningful domestic illicit production of fentanyl, although one interviewed drug policy professional recalled successful identification and disruption of two fentanyl labs in Quebec (see, e.g., "Fentanyl Found for the First Time in Illegal Quebec Drug Lab, Says SQ," 2016).

Some fentanyl on the Canadian illicit market has been diverted from the Canadian health care system. The extent of fentanyl diversion has varied across provinces, with Ontario particularly affected (Gomes et al., 2018). The contribution of fentanyl diversion to the burden of the opioid crisis has been highlighted in existing literature (e.g., Fischer, Vojtila, and Rehm, 2018), although all Canadian interviewees commenting on this topic generally agreed that it had been overshadowed by illicitly manufactured fentanyl, particularly in the past few years.

User Population, Preferences, and Harms

There are no official national estimates of the size of the illicit opioid user population in Canada. Historically, heroin use has been concentrated in British Columbia (particularly centered on Vancouver) and, to a lesser extent, in Toronto and Montreal. The number of individuals in medication treatment in 2017 was estimated at 70,000 (Eibl et al., 2017) and is plausibly higher today. Furthermore, according to a "crude estimate" developed by Fischer et al. (2018) based on population survey data, there were nearly 350,000 people with prescription opioid disorder in Canada. This number does not include users of illegal or diverted prescription opioids. In provincial estimates, based on literature review and key informant interviews, the Centre for Global Public Health (2016) estimates that there were 42,200 PWID in British Columbia in 2015. Similarly, based on administrative data, Janjua et al. (2018) estimates that there were 41,400 PWID in the province from 2013 to 2015.

---

[35] The federal government and Alberta passed pill press legislation in 2016. Other provinces passed their own legislation, which was intended to introduce regulations on top of the federal rules more recently (Province of British Columbia, Public Safety and Solicitor General, 2018). For instance, British Columbia passed its Pill Press and Related Equipment Control Act in May 2018 (Legislative Assembly of British Columbia, 2018).

The arrival of fentanyl substantially increased the number of drug-related deaths (see Table 4.3), with particularly dramatic growth in 2016 and 2017. The death rate has been the highest in British Columbia, followed by Alberta. Ontario had the third-highest death rate as of 2018, which, because of its large population, results in nearly the same absolute number as in British Columbia. Fentanyl and fentanyl-related harms appear to have first affected the western provinces before gradually spreading east.

Focusing on the most-affected jurisdiction, Figure 4.11 shows the temporal progression of the number of deaths and the death rate (for all illicit drugs) in British Columbia from 2000 to 2018. The trend line shows a marked increase in 2016 and 2017, which corresponds to the time line of the increased share of fentanyl in opioid-related deaths.

As explained by multiple public health professionals and drug policy interviewees, British Columbia users rapidly became aware of fentanyl's availability and have come to expect it when buying illicit opioids. As discussed earlier, this is reflected in the fact that "down" refers to any opioid, although users take it to mean something contain-

Table 4.3
Opioid-Related Death Rates in Canada per 100,000 People

Area	2016	2017	2018
British Columbia	20.7	30.8	30.6
Alberta	14.3	17.5	18
Saskatchewan	7.3	7.4	8.2
Manitoba	6.7	7.9	4.6
Ontario	6.2	9.0	10.3
Quebec	3.0	2.9	5.1
New Brunswick	4.3	4.8	3.5
Nova Scotia	5.6	6.7	5.9
Newfoundland	3.4	6.2	1.9
Nationwide	8.4	11.2	12
Percentage of accidental opioid deaths involving fentanyl	50	67	70

SOURCE: Special Advisory Committee on the Epidemic of Opioid Overdoses, 2019.
NOTE: Other provinces and all territories had at least one reference period with fewer than ten deaths or with suppressed data.

Figure 4.11
Illicit Drug Deaths and Death Rate in British Columbia, 2000–2018

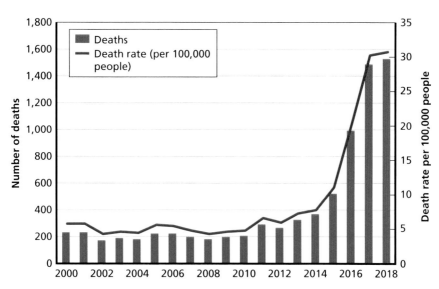

SOURCE: Data are from British Columbia Coroners Service, 2019.

ing fentanyl or another analog. A similar observation was made by a researcher involved in services for PWID in Ontario, who noted that the local user population knows that specifically asking for and obtaining "heroin" is not an option for them.

The majority of interviewees from every stakeholder group, including public health professionals working for organizations providing services to PWUD, opined that at least some users prefer fentanyl. Others (for instance, long-term heroin users) might prefer heroin but will use fentanyl if that is what is available. This is consistent with the findings of a recent survey of opioid users conducted by the British Columbia Center on Substance Use (BCCSU), in which 80 percent of respondents expressed a preference for heroin (if available), while 16 percent preferred fentanyl (BCCSU, 2019).

Current Situation

Fentanyl and its analogs continue to be the dominant cause of opioid-related harms in Canada. There is no indication that the supply of illicitly manufactured fentanyls has been disrupted, and despite intense efforts at the federal, provincial, and local levels, early projections suggest that the number of opioid-related deaths in 2018 exceeded that in 2017, although the rate of growth appears to have slowed (see, e.g., "B.C.'s Top Doctor Calls for Regulated Opioid Supply After Almost 1,500 Overdose Deaths in 2018," 2019).

Summary of Market Characteristics and Variations Across Countries

In Table 4.4, we summarize historical developments in the five focus countries and compare them with the situation in the United States.[36] The first row looks at the extent to which heroin has been replaced by other opioids. In Estonia and Finland, heroin has been fully replaced by fentanyl and its analogs and by diverted buprenorphine, respectively. In Latvia and Canada, fentanyl or fentanyl analogs have largely taken up the position previously held by heroin. By contrast, in Sweden, the fentanyl analog market established itself alongside the heroin one and remains separate.

There are strong parallels among two subsets of countries. For instance, the changes in the Estonian and Finnish drug markets took place at approximately the same time, in early 2002, soon after the Taliban's poppy ban created heroin shortages in Europe. The similarities in the time line for the appearance of fentanyl and/or analogs in the other focus countries is even more striking. In all countries, save Finland, the beginning of the large-scale presence of new synthetic opioids dates to the 2014–2015 time frame, which is identical to the United States and also corresponds with the emergence of fentanyl analogs other than 3MF in Estonia. Latvia and Canada first detected these substances earlier in the 2010s, but it would be premature to describe these detections as systemic outbreaks.

---

[36] Note that, for the North American countries, this discussion pertains to areas affected by fentanyl (i.e., primarily British Columbia, Alberta, and Ontario in Canada and the eastern half of the United States).

Table 4.4
Historical Comparison of Markets in Focus Countries

Attribute	Estonia	Finland	Latvia	Sweden	Canada (British Columbia, Alberta, Ontario)	United States (East)
Overall picture	Fentanyl has fully replaced heroin	Buprenorphine has fully replaced heroin	Analogs have increasingly replaced heroin	Fentanyl and analogs are sold alongside heroin	Fentanyl and analogs have increasingly replaced heroin in some provinces	Fentanyl and analogs have increasingly replaced heroin in certain states
Timeline of fentanyl arrival	2002 for fentanyl; 2015 for analogs	2002 for buprenorphine; nothing since	2012 for analogs (first appearance); 2015 for analogs (large-scale presence)	2014 for analogs; fentanyl diversion existed before	2012 for fentanyl and analogs (first appearance); 2015 for fentanyl and analogs (large-scale presence)	2013–2014 (first appearance); 2016 (large-scale presence)
Heroin availability	Not available since the early 2000s	Not available since the early 2000s	Decreased	Not significantly changed	Decreased since 2015	Decreased in a few places
Current situation	Availability of fentanyl severely disrupted in 2017 and 2018	Market stable	Continued dominance of fentanyl and analogs	Analog market dismantled in 2017 and 2018 and has not been replaced	Continued strong presence of fentanyl and analogs	Continued strong presence of fentanyl and analogs

The situation regarding heroin use in these five countries reflects the trends described earlier. In Estonia and Finland, heroin has been practically absent from the national markets since the early 2000s. In Latvia and Canada, heroin availability has decreased substantially since 2015, but continues to be available to a limited extent. Again, Sweden represents an exception in that the fentanyl market does not appear to have affected the availability of heroin and, remarkably, the two markets remain separate.

The current situations in Finland, Latvia, and Canada appear to represent a continuation of the trends described earlier, marked by the dominance of either buprenorphine (Finland) or fentanyl and its analogs (Latvia and Canada). By contrast, Estonia and Sweden saw significant market changes in recent years, at least partially as a result of law enforcement operations against fentanyl traffickers in both countries. In Sweden, the fentanyl analog market appears to have been fully dismantled through efforts to target local distributors, while in Estonia, the market has been severely disrupted, with recorded decreases in fentanyl availability and concomitant harms.

The fentanyl markets in the focus countries also vary in some of their characteristics (see Table 4.5). China is thought to be the current source of illicitly manufactured fentanyl and analogs for all four focus countries with fentanyl markets. In addition, Russia is considered to have been a source of fentanyl in Estonia, although the extent to which this has continued to be the case is unclear. Diversions from the domestic health care sector were reported in Canada and Sweden, although in neither instance as significantly as was illicitly manufactured fentanyl. Minimal volume of domestic fentanyl diversion is also present in Latvia and Estonia. No country in the sample has seen major domestic production of fentanyl, although illicit fentanyl laboratories were identified and dismantled in Canada and Estonia. Fentanyl and fentanyl analogs are generally imported as powder, but Estonian law enforcement interviewees also recalled the possibility of fentanyl smuggled from Russia in a liquid form and turned into powder in Estonia. Injecting is the main form of administration, except in Sweden, where the dominant form has been nasal sprays (individuals who inject drugs continue to be served by a separate heroin market). In Canada, and, to

International Experiences with Synthetic Opioids   105

Table 4.5
Comparison of Fentanyl Market Characteristics in Focus Countries

Attribute	Estonia	Finland	Latvia	Sweden	Canada (British Columbia, Alberta, Ontario)	United States (East)
Principal source of fentanyl or analogs	Russia (fentanyl), China (analogs)	N/A	China	Sweden (diverted prescription), China (analogs)	China (illicit), Canada (diverted prescription)	China (analogs and fentanyl), Mexico (fentanyl)
Diversion of licit fentanyl	Minimal	Not reported	Minimal	Yes	Yes	Yes
Domestic production	Minimal	N/A	No	No	Minimal	Unlikely or unclear, although pill pressing occurs
Import formulation	Powder from China; liquid from Russia	N/A	Powder from China	Powder from China	Powder from China	Powder from China or Mexico; pills from Mexico and, to a lesser extent, Canada
Route of administration most commonly reported	Mainly injecting	N/A	Mainly injecting	Nasal spray (analogs); smoking (patches)	Mainly injecting	Unknown
Counterfeit pills	No	No	No	Limited	Yes	Yes
Fentanyl found in or with heroin?	No	N/A	Yes	No	Yes	Yes

a much smaller extent, in Sweden, fentanyl also has been pressed into counterfeit prescription tablets, which can be crushed and injected.

In Canada and Latvia, seizures containing both fentanyl or analogs and heroin have been reported, although they are no longer common, given the decreased availability of heroin. Neither Estonia nor Sweden have seen this phenomenon; heroin is practically non-existent in Estonia and there is no link between the heroin and fentanyl markets in Sweden. All countries with fentanyl have reported a limited number of instances in which fentanyl or analogs have been found in nonopioids, such as cocaine or methamphetamine. In Sweden, fentanyl analogs have been found in counterfeit Xanax tablets containing benzodiazepines. Swedish law enforcement interviewees offered mixed perspectives on the origins of this phenomenon; some opined that this was a result of intentional mixing by dealers, while others felt that this was a product of their inadvertent contamination.

Although it would be insightful to compare the fentanyl-related mortality rate among PWUD in these five countries, it is an extremely difficult task for multiple reasons. First, there might be considerable variation in the accuracy of mortality data, with different countries employing different postmortem toxicology screens. More importantly, data collection methods, definitions, and the scope of data collection vary across countries (see, e.g., Kilmer, Reuter, and Giommoni, 2015; and Noor, Singleton, and Kalamara, 2018, for a discussion of methodological challenges). With respect to the size of the user population, the scope of the estimates varies. In most countries, the user population refers to PWID, but in Sweden, it refers to users of illicit opioids irrespective of the mode of administration. Similarly, most countries report the overall number of deaths, most of which pertain to opioids, but Sweden provides drug-specific deaths, although there could be some overlap across categories because the data note only the presence of the drug in the deceased person, irrespective of any causality considerations. These caveats limit direct comparability across countries.

Table 4.6 presents data about PWUD and mortality for the five countries, but we strongly caution against using these data to make

Table 4.6
Estimates of People Who Use Drugs and Those Who Died of Fatal Overdose in Five Countries

Factor	Estonia (2017)	Finland (2017)	Sweden: Heroin (2017)	Sweden: Heroin and Fentanyl (2017)	Latvia (2017)	British Columbia (2017)
Estimated user population	8,400 (PWID)	14,000 (high-risk opioid users)	5,000 (heroin users)	6,000 (heroin and fentanyl users)	7,000 (high-risk opioid users)	42,000 (PWID)
Number of deaths	110 (total)	200 (total)	97 (heroin)	238 (heroin and fentanyl)	22 (total)	1,500 (total)

SOURCES: Estonia: user population (EMCDDA, 2019a), deaths (Statistics Estonia, 2019); Finland: user population and deaths (EMCDDA, 2019b); Sweden: user population and deaths (Polisen, 2018); Latvia: user population and deaths (EMCDDA, 2019c); British Columbia: user population (Centre for Global Public Health, 2016), deaths (British Columbia Coroners Service, 2019).
NOTES: We strongly caution against using these data to make comparisons about mortality rates.

comparisons about mortality rates. For most countries, we present the latest available data, but we focus on 2017 data for Estonia and Sweden in order to capture the state of the market before significant law enforcement–led disruptions took place. For Sweden, we list separately the heroin market only (reflecting its stand-alone position) as well as a combined indicator of heroin and fentanyl.

Factors Associated with the Emergence of Fentanyl

As we discussed in the previous section, the evolution and characteristics of fentanyl markets in different jurisdictions have varied markedly. In this section, we identify commonalities as well as points of divergence that might shed light on factors that could be associated with the emergence of fentanyl. The available evidence does not enable us to say that a given factor is sufficient or even necessary for fentanyl to arrive in a particular market. The aspiration here is merely to identify conditions in which fentanyl tends to appear.

Existence of an Established Opioid User Population

In all countries, fentanyl and related substances have largely served an already existing opioid user population. These substances either displace a previously used opioid and/or fill a supply gap (see the section on "Disruption in Supply of 'Traditional' Opioids"). Typically, the displaced opioid was heroin, although, as interviewees pointed out, at least some fentanyl users in Canada and Sweden have likely never been heroin users; rather, they previously used prescription opioids.

In none of the countries in our sample did the arrival of fentanyl lead to a notable increase in the size of the opioid user population. In Latvia and Estonia, interviewee testimonies and existing estimates (where available) generally point to a continuing decline in the population that does not appear to have changed much with the introduction of fentanyl or its analogs. This is despite the fact that the arrival of fentanyl and analogs led to a reduction in the effective price of opioids, suggesting that fentanyl is not an attractive drug for initiation. In Sweden, a few law enforcement interviewees suggested that the establishment of the fentanyl analog market could have led to the recruitment of some opioid-naïve users (e.g., users of other new psychoactive substances), but these new users are not considered to account for a large share of the analog market (Polisen, 2018). In Canada, there are no regularly produced series of national or provincial estimates of the prevalence of opioid use and, therefore, it is difficult to assess trends; however, there is no evidence to suggest that the arrival of fentanyl and related substances has resulted in a notable increase in the number of opioid users.

Disruption in Supply of "Traditional" Opioids

In several countries, fentanyl emerged after a disruption in the supply of "traditional" opioids. For example, fentanyl became dominant in Estonia following a severe shortage of heroin in the early 2000s. At the same time, existing connections between Russian-speaking organized crime groups in Estonia and Russian sources were highlighted by several interviewees as instrumental in bringing fentanyl to the Estonian market.[37] Canada offers a different example. As several public health and law enforcement interviewees pointed out, there was no shortage of heroin in the run-up to the fentanyl outbreak in 2014. In fact, user survey data from British Columbia suggest that the perceived availability of heroin increased between 2010 and 2014 (Ho et al., 2018). Instead, change in Canada took the form of restrictions on legal prescribing of pharmaceutical opioids, which prompted users to seek diverted pharmaceuticals or other substances on the illicit market. The illicit market became increasingly dominated by fentanyl and related substances, in the form of either counterfeit pain reliever tablets (earlier on) or powder (currently). This shift could have been precipitated by the adoption of pill press legislation in Canada, as well as the possibility that the counterfeit nature of the pills became generally known among users, obviating the need for deception.

Latvia offers two insights pertaining to disruptions in supply. One law enforcement interviewee pointed out that the arrival of carfentanil in the country in 2012 took place amid a shortage of heroin, as evidenced by decreasing purity and users' reports of lower availability.[38] In addition, Latvia offers an interesting contrast with Estonia with respect to the situation in the early 2000s, when Estonia's opioid market was overtaken by fentanyl, while heroin remained dominant in Latvia. One interviewee suggested that a possible explanation for this difference is that Latvian dealer networks managed to ensure at least some continu-

---

[37] The same suggestion was made in academic literature. Although data are scarce, evidence documents the existence of fentanyl in western Russia in the late 1990s and well into the 2000s. (Ojanpera et al., 2008). However, it is not clear how long the fentanyl presence in Russia lasted. For instance, Uusküla et al. (2015) examined risk factors among PWID in Kohtla-Jarve (northeast Estonia) and in St. Petersburg and found that in 2012 and 2013, almost no users in St. Petersburg reported fentanyl as their main injected drug.

[38] The interviewee acknowledged the existence of an opposing view held by others monitoring the situation in Latvia, which claims that heroin was displaced from the market after the introduction of carfentanil. However, according to the interviewee, this view does not appear to be supported by indicators, such as purity, or user testimonies. Decreases in heroin availability in the early 2010s were also noted in the 2018 European Drug Report (based on 2016 data), which noted an overall drop in heroin seizures in multiple countries (EMCDDA 2018d).

ity of heroin supply, which helped the market weather the temporary shortage in the early 2000s.

This observation is also consistent with Mounteney et al. (2015), which describes the emergence of fentanyl in several countries facing a heroin shortage. Hempstead and Yildirim (2014) makes a similar point regarding the situation in New Jersey in connection with the fentanyl outbreak in 2006, although other factors discussed in the previous chapter also could have played a role.

User Preferences and Habits

Interviewees in all countries referred to local user preferences when explaining fentanyl's market trajectory, regardless of whether that country had much fentanyl.

To illustrate this point, every interviewee commenting on the Finnish market (spanning law enforcement, public health, and drug policy professionals) noted that Finnish users are not interested in fentanyl and believed that that might help explain why it has never appeared on a large scale in the country. Users' experiences with buprenorphine and its image as a safer and more predictable drug, combined with its unimpeded availability, contributed to diverted buprenorphine, rather than fentanyl, replacing heroin in the early 2000s.[39]

However, users' preferences were also cited as reasons why fentanyl gained and kept a dominant position in other countries. One drug policy professional commenting on Estonia noted that when fentanyl arrived on a large scale in the early 2000s, it delivered a stronger high and was cheaper than other alternatives, such as buprenorphine. Multiple interviewees generally agreed that, over time, Estonian users became tolerant to fentanyl and would probably not be interested in a weaker alternative (such as heroin). One interviewee noted, based on their interviews with Latvian users, that at least some users in the country were no longer interested in heroin.

---

[39] The first regulation of medication treatment with buprenorphine in Finland was published in 1997. However, buprenorphine had been prescribed by a small number of physicians before official policy was adopted, leading to high-profile policy and practice discussions, which in turn raised the profile of buprenorphine as an option for heavy drug users (Selin et al., 2013).

Users' preferences also were cited in Sweden, and in both directions. In particular, users' reluctance to embrace fentanyl was cited by a law enforcement interviewee as a possible contributing reason for why the street-level fentanyl introduced in Sweden in 2002 disappeared after 2004. Referring to developments a decade later, however, another law enforcement interviewee suggested that Sweden's long tradition of new psychoactive substance use, along with online sales, facilitated the emergence of the online fentanyl analog marketplace.

Themes Emerging from Existing Fentanyl Markets

Interviewees also commented on other themes or notable features of fentanyl-dominated drug markets that have been observed in at least some focus countries and bear some commonalities across jurisdictions.

General Lack of Information Among Buyers and Sellers

Across all focus countries with fentanyl markets, interviewees from all stakeholder groups stressed that users often do not know what they are buying, either in terms of composition or potency. This is not necessarily a new feature of drug markets, but the range of potency offered by a variety of synthetic opioids greatly exacerbates the risks stemming from the use of street drugs in markets dominated by fentanyl and its analogs. In Canada and Latvia, users are faced with the possibility that what they are buying is any of the following: (1) fentanyl or an analog only, (2) fentanyl or an analog mixed with heroin, or (3) heroin only.[40] This dilemma is further exacerbated by the proliferation of fentanyl analogs, which substantially increases the possible number of substances available. In Estonia and Sweden, where the mixing of heroin with fentanyl has not been documented, users are aware that they are

---

[40] A 2015 study from British Columbia (Amlani et al., 2015) concluded that, based on a comparison of urine samples and users' self-reports, a large portion of fentanyl use might be unintentional. However, it is plausible that, with the increases in the availability of fentanyl and its displacement of heroin, users at least know that there is a strong possibility that their purchased sample will include fentanyl.

purchasing fentanyl or its analogs but still cannot be certain about which analog is present or how potent the sample is.[41]

Importantly, interviewees in all countries added that sellers also lack information about what they are selling, particularly if they are far removed from the original synthesis or manufacturing process. This is similar to the situation in the United States (Mars, Rosenblum, and Ciccarone, 2018).

Drug-checking services provide hard data on the gap between what users *think* they bought and what they *actually* bought. From October 2017 to April 2018, one drug-checking service run by the BCCSU and Vancouver Coastal Health analyzed 907 samples that buyers expected to be heroin. In reality, only 17.6 percent of these samples contained any heroin, but more than 90 percent tested positive for fentanyl (Tupper et al., 2018). This illustrates the uncertainty present in the market, although, as several interviewees noted, the meaning of users' traditional street references for heroin has evolved to the point where slang terms might refer to any illicit opioid, including fentanyl.[42]

Limited Detection Capabilities and Data on Markets

Interviewees from every country commented that, while they are improving, data on markets with fentanyl and related substances continue to be patchy. One contributing factor is limitations in detection capabilities, which might hamper understanding of the fentanyl phenomenon and its historical development. To illustrate this point, one interviewee pointed out that, prior to the current opioid crisis in Canada, British Columbia experienced several waves (around 1997 and 2011) of what people interpreted as very potent heroin; in reality, this

---

[41] Analogs in Sweden are marketed as such, but there is no guarantee that buyers will receive the declared substance. Swedish seizures have identified cases of erroneous labels.

[42] Again, this is similar to the situation in the past in the United States with the reported use of the ambiguous term "China White," which could have referred to synthetic opioids or Southeast Asian heroin (Hibbs, Perper, and Winek, 1991; Mars, Rosenblum, and Ciccarone, 2018).

could have been heroin spiked with fentanyl, but the province lacked the capability to detect fentanyl and its analogs.[43]

According to multiple interviewees, the emergence of novel fentanyl analogs poses a particular problem. Novel compounds might avoid detection by public health surveillance systems and law enforcement, and drug-checking services might not be able to provide an answer to their clients who use drugs because the chemicals in question are not yet included in the reference library used by the analytical technology. Elsewhere, the collection of important indicators and variables might not be possible. For instance, one Latvian interviewee noted that the country's surveillance system only checks for the presence of particular compounds and does not monitor purity. In addition to counts, most data on seizures report information only on one dimension: weight. This leaves out data on purity, which represent an essential component in characterizing supply, in particular because fentanyl and fentanyl analogs are dosed in minute quantities.

Market Adjustments and Learning

Trend data and interview testimonies suggest that the emergence of fentanyl and/or its analogs tends to be followed by a period of market adjustment and learning on the part of market participants. This process involves users learning to dose and use more safely, as well as dealers learning how to cut and market the new product. This initial adjustment might result in a relatively stable period of equilibrium until the market is disrupted by the arrival of a new substance.

To illustrate, in Estonia, since 2002, the number of drug-related deaths spiked immediately after the arrival of a new substance (e.g., fentanyl, 3MF, other analogs), but then edged back. Along similar lines, one interviewee in Canada recalled that the emergence of carfentanil in British Columbia in 2016 resulted in a dramatic increase in the number of deaths and emergency room episodes. However, after

---

[43] The product on the market during the 1997 outbreak in British Columbia was referred to as "China White." An emergence of "China White" in California in the 1980s was subsequently confirmed to have been 3MF, leading the interviewee to believe that the same product might have been present in British Columbia as well.

a period of time, the number of overdoses decreased, even though the number of screens testing positive for carfentanil continued to grow. In another example, one law enforcement interviewee commenting on Latvia recalled how the arrival of carfentanil was similarly followed by a notable increase in the number of deaths. After some time, the number of deaths went down, even though the number of emergency medical services episodes stayed elevated. This suggests that users were able to find a way to use carfentanil relatively more safely.[44] Importantly, the drug-related death rate in Latvia continues to be relatively low, particularly for a country with an analog-dominated market, and the rate is not higher than it was in the years before the arrival of fentanyl analogs, although the size of the user population has decreased over time.[45] This suggests that it is possible for fentanyl markets to adjust in a way that does not translate into substantial permanent increases in mortality over heroin-dominated markets seen in other jurisdictions.

Persistence of Fentanyl and Its Future

Experience from international markets suggests that fentanyl has the potential to stay in a prominent position in countries' drug markets,

---

[44] See, e.g., Ciccarone, Ondocsin, and Mars (2017) for a discussion of possible harm-reduction strategies employed by users in markets undergoing transition from heroin to fentanyl. Similarly, Mars, Ondocsin, and Ciccarone (2018b) shows how opioid users can use drug-sampling methods to minimize risks.

[45] According to an interviewed drug policy professional, there is no evidence-based explanation for the relatively low death rate in Latvia, particularly in comparison with neighboring Estonia. One potential factor suggested by the interviewee was the fact that the use of fentanyl is concentrated in cities, allowing for rapid emergency response. Another possibility is new fentanyls going undetected in autopsies, which would produce an undercount of the true number of drug-related deaths. This interviewee added that this explanation is tentatively supported by police information on several death cases, which, according to law enforcement operational information, were fatal overdoses but were not confirmed as such in autopsies. This possible cause of underreporting also was mentioned in the EMCDDA Statistical Bulletin, along with reductions in funding, which could result in a lower number of deceased people examined, as well as possible issues with death definition for young adults (EMCDDA, 2019e). The results of a recent cohort study of high-risk individuals in Latvia suggested that some drug overdoses went unrecognized in the country's general mortality register (EMCDDA, 2019g). Still, the extent of undercounting would have to be very substantial for the death rate to reach Estonian levels because the death rate among the user population in Estonia is estimated to be multiples of that in Latvia (see Table 4.6).

although Estonia remains the only existing example of a long-term fentanyl market to date. In Estonia, Latvia, and affected Canadian provinces alike, fentanyl and its analogs have taken over a position previously occupied by heroin—completely in Estonia and to a substantial extent in Latvia and Canada.[46] Individual analogs might come and go, but they have tended to be replaced by other new synthetic opioids. In other cases, fentanyl remains dominant in seizure and death data.

Interviewees also were invited to comment on expected future trends. Key informants from every country with a fentanyl market agreed that new synthetic opioids are likely here to stay. A few interviewees highlighted the advantages that fentanyl and its analogs offer to organized criminal groups and noted that there were no market incentives for distributors to move away from new synthetic opioids.[47]

Recent developments in Estonia and Sweden have demonstrated that some fentanyl markets can be successfully disrupted, although any lessons from these two countries need to be put into perspective. The Estonian fentanyl market is not large in absolute terms and its distribution networks were, until recently, dominated by very few key players.[48] This means that even relatively small supply-side interventions can have a sizable effect.[49] According to the accounts of interviewees with familiarity of the cases, the operations by Estonian law enforcement in 2017 focused on taking out a small number of key individuals. This was successful in temporarily disrupting the supply of fentanyl. The emergence of new distribution groups and some increase in

---

[46] The province of Quebec might be an exception to this observation because the share of opioid deaths involving fentanyl decreased from 2016 to 2018. The burden of the opioid crisis in Quebec is, however, notably lower than in British Columbia, Alberta, and Ontario, which account for the majority of Canadian opioid-related deaths.

[47] See Chapter Five for a discussion of possible disadvantages of fentanyl to drug traffickers. Although this issue was not raised by any interviewees, one such risk could be the loss of customers due to increased deaths.

[48] A quick calculation, assuming 5,000 fentanyl users, a dose of 2 mg of pure fentanyl, and four injections per day puts the annual consumption of pure fentanyl at nearly 15 kg.

[49] Of course, this does not detract from the overarching challenge discussed in Chapter Three; if comparatively smaller quantities are necessary to supply a market, it makes it more difficult to detect and interdict these shipments.

the availability of fentanyl have been reported, albeit not to levels seen before the 2017 takedowns, and the Estonian market remains in flux.

Sweden offers a similar lesson in that its online analog market was shut down following the targeted prosecution of its three biggest players. According to law enforcement interviewees, mounting such a successful operation was possible because, as was the case in Estonia, the number of vendors selling analogs in Sweden was very limited, unlikely exceeding 15. As one interviewee suggested, a disruption of this scale would have been impossible if fentanyl analogs had been distributed in a less concentrated way or as part of the street-level market, as they were in Estonia. Unlike in Estonia, there has been no sign of a comeback in Sweden so far.

Reflections on Lessons for the United States from Other Countries

This examination of fentanyl markets in the selected focus countries demonstrates the variability in the form these markets can take. Indicators of interest in this regard include basic characteristics, such as the extent of mixing fentanyl with heroin, availability of fentanyl analogs, and their number. This is not dissimilar to differences among individual U.S. states, some of which have been dominated by fentanyl (New Hampshire), by fentanyl analogs (Ohio), or which continue to have a mix of fentanyl and heroin (Kentucky). Therefore, just as we discuss variability across international jurisdictions (including countries adjacent or very close to each other), it would be inaccurate to speak of a homogeneous U.S. fentanyl market.

The historical developments of the Canadian fentanyl market are the most relevant for comparisons with the United States, primarily because of the existence of a prescription opioid crisis in both countries. The Canadian experience also is comparable in terms of recent trends and growth in the severity of the issue. Consequently, the Canadian response to the emergence of fentanyl and associated policy discussions could offer relevant lessons for the United States, although there are notable differences in the delivery of public health and social services between the two countries.

In contrast, after decades of heroin dominating high-risk drug use in Europe, the many different European experiences with fentanyl described here take place in the context of generally decreasing opioid use, with relatively few new users entering the market. In addition, although the nonprescribed use of prescription opioids—in particular, tramadol—has been noted as a concern in some of the focus countries, the extent of the phenomenon is not comparable with the situation in North America. For that reason, the etiology of fentanyl issues in Europe could offer lessons primarily for jurisdictions that have not yet experienced a major synthetic opioid issue.

For the North American context, the European experience might offer insights into potential future issues and trends. To illustrate, Estonia offers an indication of what an established, mature fentanyl market might look like more than a decade after the introduction of synthetic opioids. Latvia provides an example of a market that skipped the fentanyl phase and proceeded directly to a phase dominated by more-powerful fentanyl analogs, which, as far as the available data suggest, is a scenario not seen in any North American jurisdiction so far. Notably, this transition has failed to result in substantial permanent increases in drug-related deaths in the country. Thus, for the purposes of future U.S. projections, Latvia suggests that it is possible to have market adjustments where dominance by synthetic opioids does not automatically equate to much higher death rates. Furthermore, Sweden demonstrates the possibility of having a fentanyl market with a novel product (e.g., nasal sprays) that is in a unique relationship with the heroin market (i.e., completely separate), with novel modes of distribution and marketing (e.g., the sprays are sold as fentanyl analogs online to end users). Again, none of these three features has been observed in the United States to a notable extent.

Lastly, it is worth adding that one area in which international experience might not yet be in a position to offer lessons to the United States is the potential threat of fentanyl contaminating other drug markets, in particular stimulants. Methamphetamine, rather than cocaine, is an issue in the European countries included in this analysis; however, these markets do not seem to be fentanyl-affected to a meaning-ful extent. Similarly, the presence of fentanyl and its analogs in the Canadian cocaine market, while documented, appears to be limited.[50]

---

[50] According to Drug Analysis Service data cited in Miller and Ireland (2017), in 2016, fentanyl was detected in 1.8 percent of submitted cocaine samples. According to newer Drug Analysis Service data provided to the research team that cover May 2018 to March 2019, synthetic opioids were found in approximately 7 percent of all submitted cocaine samples.

CHAPTER FIVE

Some Possible Futures for Fentanyl and Other Synthetic Opioids

Based on the previous analyses and interviews, we outline some possible future scenarios for fentanyl and other synthetic opioids. Our intent is not to predict but rather to provide a framework for thinking about potential trajectories for these substances' market positions. Our premise is that, with respect to fentanyl and other synthetic opioids, drug markets are in flux rather than in equilibrium, and the long run might not be a simple extrapolation of recent trends. We liken this exercise to predicting the future of aviation in 1903, immediately after Orville and Wilbur Wright's flight, or the future of cell phones in 2007, the year the iPhone was introduced. This chapter indulges in thought experiments rooted in basic facts about fentanyl and general wisdom about drug markets, not just extrapolation of existing data series.

One reason for market expansion is that fentanyl is phenomenally inexpensive per dose in wholesale markets. In Appendix B, we assemble data suggesting that fentanyl's import price per MED is 1 percent or less than that of heroin. The same might be true for wholesale transactions within the United States. For example, Bosio, Mignone, and Norio (2018) mentions an undercover purchase of 1 kg of fentanyl for $3,800 versus $50,000 per kilogram for heroin. Assuming that it takes about 20 g of heroin to produce the same number of MEDs as 1 g of fentanyl, that particular price snapshot would make heroin more than 250 times as expensive per MED.[1]

Bosio, Mignone, and Norio (2018) suggests several other reasons why the fentanyl market could expand, including the following: (1) high potency is attractive to users who have developed tolerance, despite the obvious overdose risk (Ciccarone, Ondocsin, and Mars, 2017); (2) chemists can produce new analogs that are not yet banned in all jurisdictions; and (3) suppliers not affiliated with traditional DTOs can easily enter the market. Concerning the last point, the ability to order drugs over the internet for delivery by mail means that local wholesale dealers do not need to source from violent organized crime groups or provide the resources and capacity needed to smuggle material across international borders.

We describe four potential scenarios for fentanyl's market position a decade hence. We then add some thoughts about how fentanyl's expansion might affect drug-related crime and violence if it substantially displaces heroin. The scenarios are not mutually exclusive, and different ones could persist in different regions for extended periods. In Chapter Four, we described such heterogeneity across Estonia, Finland, Sweden, and Latvia. The discussion in this chapter points toward fentanyl pushing heroin out of at least an important subset of opioid markets, but we close by discussing several possibilities that might offset fentanyl's cost advantage and moderate its growth.

Scenario 1: Flash and Recede

There is no question that fentanyl's presence in drug markets has grown exponentially, but some things that go up do come down again. Indeed, fentanyl itself did that in California in the early 1980s (Henderson, 1988) and again at a larger scale from 2005 to 2007 (CDC, 2008). There also have been several small outbreaks in Europe that

---

[1]   Bosio, Mignone, and Norio (2018) does not report purities, but wholesale amounts of fentanyl imported from China are purer than wholesale imports of heroin, so the differential in cost per MED could be larger.

did not have staying power (Mounteney, Evans-Brown, and Giraudon, 2012).

However, synthetic opioids disappearing, or largely disappearing, seems unlikely. The international and past U.S. experience is that *small* fentanyl markets might pop up and recede, but there is no recorded instance of synthetic opioids reaching a dominant market position in a market and then withering away. Furthermore, fentanyl is now produced in many labs, not just in one as from 2005 to 2007, and its cost advantages are too enormous for unscrupulous drug dealers to set aside (see Appendix B). It is possible that fentanyl has yet to peak in the United States. As we observed in Chapter Two, large swaths of the country have not yet been fully exposed to the degree that New England, Ohio, and West Virginia have.

That said, some reduction in severity after a peak would not be surprising; that pattern is a recurring theme in drug epidemics (Caulkins, 2005). Musto (1999) argues that drug epidemics ebb when the drug's dangers become widely known. The fact that a negative reputation could tamp down initiation was observed with cocaine in the latter years of both the 19th and 20th centuries. For example, cocaine initiation declined around the time that the 1986 deaths of Len Bias and Don Rogers poignantly illustrated that cocaine can strike down even paragons of physical fitness (Everingham, Rydell, and Caulkins, 1995).

However, the dynamics of fentanyl use seem different from those of a prototypical drug epidemic. Fentanyl and other synthetic opioids do not generate a wave of drug initiation among youth or even necessarily stimulate greater demand more generally; interviewees in Europe noted that opioids already had a bad reputation among nonusers. Rather, it appears to spread primarily among existing users when suppliers substitute fentanyl for another drug (to date, another opioid). This triggers a wave of deaths mostly by increasing lethality (deaths per person-year of use), rather than by increasing the number of users. Indeed, the number of individuals who inject drugs in Estonia peaked in the late 1990s, several years *before* fentanyl's arrival, and fentanyl might even deter longtime opioid users. Carroll and colleagues (2017, p. 142) reports that some opioid users "explicitly described a frighten-

ing encounter with fentanyl as directly responsible for their treatment seeking."

Musto (1999) imagines a diffuse, societywide learning that leads to rejection of a dangerous drug, but another variant of this theory is proactive self-policing by user groups. Gilbert and Dasgupta (2017) reports that the invitation-only cryptomarket Darknet Heroes League decided to ban the sale of fentanyl and its analogs in 2016, and apparently user forums actively discuss the ethical responsibility of market operators to ban such dangerous drugs. In the past, online distribution has captured only a small share of all sales, limiting the scope of internet-mediated self-policing, but online distribution might gain a larger share of the market in the future.

An optimist might hope that prudent policy could promote such societal learning. Although skepticism about the ability of scare tactics to prevent drug use is the norm (Substance Abuse and Mental Health Service Administration [SAMHSA], 2015), meta-analyses of fear appeals in social marketing find that they can induce behavior change (e.g., Tannenbaum et al., 2015), and there could be a difference between the public's response to sensational exaggeration of the risks of cannabis and dry reporting of fentanyl's death toll.

In theory, the use of synthetic opioids might recede if their supply gets curtailed. As we discussed in Chapter Four, Estonia (temporarily) and Sweden (perhaps permanently) disrupted fentanyl supply chains by taking down key distributors. Law enforcement also is credited with shutting down the 2005–2007 outbreak in the United States. That, however, was associated with a single lab in Mexico, creating a single point of vulnerability; today, there are many producers and online sellers in China, which does not have the same history of or incentives for cooperating with U.S. law enforcement as does Mexico (Humphreys, Caulkins, and Felbab-Brown, 2018; Pardo, Kilmer, and Huang, 2019). Furthermore, all three of those successes came against much smaller markets. Achieving something similar could be unlikely today.[2]

---

[2]   Another possibility is imposing tougher sentences for importing and distributing fentanyl than for other substances. In theory, this might encourage self-interested dealers to sell less-dangerous drugs through a sort of harm-reduction version of supply control (Caulkins and

Scenario 2: Synthetic Opioids Added to the Drug Mix

Fentanyl cuts heroin dealers' raw materials costs by more than 99 percent. The cost advantage for dealers of counterfeit pills is also striking. Fentanyl's MED is 50–100 versus 1.5 for oxycodone, so a dose equivalent to a 30 mg oxycodone pill would only require 0.5–1 mg of fentanyl.[3] If online vendors sell 50 g of fentanyl to dealers for $500, that is just one penny per milligram, and dealers can sell a 30 mg oxycodone pill—or its counterfeit equivalent—for $20 on the black market.[4]

Thus, even if customers never ask for fentanyl by name, they might still get it in street bags and fake pills that contain other drugs, or at least are advertised as such. After all, drug dealers' wares are not subject to regulatory oversight or quality control by government inspectors.

This is already happening in many markets in Canada and east of the Mississippi River in the United States, so this scenario is just a stabilization of the status quo or an extension to other regions that have not yet been as exposed to fentanyl. This scenario comes in several variants, depending on what substance(s) get adulterated:

- **Variant 2a: Fentanyl remains geographically restricted,**[5] for example, because it is used to adulterate only heroin powder

---

Reuter, 2009). Hrymak (2018) reports (disapprovingly) that even British Columbia—one of the leaders in harm-reduction approaches to drug policy—set the sentence for street-level sellers of fentanyl at "18 [to] 36 months and possibly higher" versus six to 18 months for other Schedule I substances. Sweden's crackdown included prosecuting an analog vendor for involuntary manslaughter. However, long sentences are generally seen as less effective than measures that increase the certainty of sanction (Nagin, 2013), and retail sellers might not even know that they are selling fentanyl in heroin (Reuter and Caulkins, 2004; Mars, Rosenblum, and Ciccarone, 2018).

[3]   Gilbert and Dasgupta (2017) gives an example of an online vendor that sells oxycodone pills advertised as containing 0.8 mg of fentanyl. This is an instance in which the vendor is openly reporting the fentanyl.

[4]   Per personal communication with law enforcement officers.

[5]   There are precedents for fentanyl remaining geographically constrained. It dominated in Estonia for many years without affecting its European Union neighbors. With regard to the first U.S. outbreak, of the first 110 fentanyl-related deaths that began in December 1979, all but two were in California (Henderson, 1988).

rather than the Mexican "black tar" heroin that dominates in the western United States.[6]

- **Variant 2b: Fentanyl adulterates heroin throughout the United States and Canada,** either because drug dealers succeed in mixing fentanyl into black tar heroin or because powder heroin augmented with fentanyl displaces black tar from the market.[7]
- **Variant 2c: Fentanyl is increasingly sold as counterfeit pills,** not just as heroin, expanding its reach to people who use prescription opioid pills inappropriately but who do not use heroin.
- **Variant 2d: Dealers routinely add fentanyl to stimulants.** This practice could be particularly deadly because even long-term stimulant use does not confer tolerance for opioids. (As we describe in Chapter Two, fentanyl already appears with cocaine, albeit rarely, but it is not clear whether that will persist or even how often it is intentional mixing as opposed to inadvertent contamination.)

For any of these variations, one can ask whether adding fentanyl will increase or reduce the size of the market, for various measures of market size. Consumption of many illegal drugs responds to changes in price, but less than proportionately (Gallet, 2014). By focusing only on the idea that fentanyl could reduce the cost per dose, one might expect greater use but lower total spending.

There could be other effects, though. Fentanyl also increases nondollar costs of use, notably the risk of death and disease.[8] As Moore (1977) argues, all other things being equal, increasing nondollar costs of use should reduce both use and spending. An additional effect is

---

[6] It is not clear how easily or even whether fentanyl can be mixed with black tar heroin. Lupick (2018) gives a journalistic account of why California has largely been spared by fentanyl so far and cites people saying that it is physically hard to mix a fine white powder into black tar. That said, the DEA (2016b, p. 69) has identified a tar-like substance that does contain fentanyl, but not heroin.

[7] There is a claim that "China White" (fentanyl) is starting to displace black tar in Tijuana because of its cost advantage (Debruyne, 2019).

[8] Fentanyl is shorter-acting than heroin, leading some users to inject more often per day, and, all other things being equal, this might be expected to increase the risk of spreading blood-borne infections, such as HIV.

through mortality. If fentanyl increased the death rate for chronic users from 1 percent to 4 percent per year (to use some arbitrary numbers for illustrative purposes), then that alone could cut the number of heavy users by one-quarter over a decade. That combination of considerations sums to ambiguous effects on both consumption and spending, although it seems plausible that the price declines could be large enough to produce declines in spending, even if use increases.

Scenario 3: Fewer Poppies Through Chemistry

Some heroin suppliers already embrace fentanyl. With it, they can cheaply turn one bag of 40-percent pure heroin into two bags that are 20-percent heroin plus enough fentanyl to make each of the new bags contain as many MEDs as the first bag did. But if a little fentanyl is good, why not put twice as much of it in the bag and skip the heroin altogether? From the perspective of minimizing the cost of materials, one could imagine fentanyl driving heroin and other poppy-based opioids out of the illicit market entirely.

As we discussed in Chapter Four, fentanyl displaced heroin in Estonia, and there are signs that at least some Canadian and U.S. markets might be moving in that direction. In Vancouver, a drug-checking program at a supervised consumption site found that the majority of samples that were tested came back positive for fentanyl (Karamouzian et al., 2018), and interviewees there confirmed that heroin is increasingly rare.[9] What is striking is the apparent speed of the changeover. Jones et al. (2018) reports rapid changes in fentanyl detection in urine collected in a longitudinal study of a high-risk community sample in Vancouver over five months from March 1, 2017, to July 31, 2017. By

---

[9] Of the samples tested before consumption, 76.5 percent tested positive for fentanyl, as did 82.9 percent of those tested after consumption. Because 113 of the 654 instances of post-consumption testing involved an overdose, those 654 are most likely not representative of all samples consumed at the supervised consumption site. Indeed, because only about 1 percent of visits resulted in a drug test, even the preconsumption tests might not be representative of the overall market.

the end of that period, fentanyl was detected in the urine of every respondent who reported nonprescribed opioid use.

Consider also the mortality data we explored in Chapter Two. In New Hampshire, there are now more than ten times as many overdose deaths involving synthetic opioids as those involving heroin (more than 30 per 100,000 people for synthetic opioids versus 2.4 per 100,000 people for heroin). Even if synthetic opioids produced ten times as many deaths per unit of use, that would still suggest greater use of synthetic opioids than of heroin.

Relative to Ohio, New Hampshire never had as much of a heroin market (See Chapter Two). Yet, in Ohio, fatal overdoses involving heroin increased through 2016 but fell in 2017 (to about nine per 100,000), even though deaths from synthetic opioids were still rising sharply. If fentanyl were only appearing in bags that also contained heroin, then overdose mentions for heroin should have continued to increase, not begun to decline. There also are anecdotal reports of Mexican poppy farmers saying that the market prices paid for their products are falling, in some cases by more than 80 percent (see Appendix B).

None of these observations is decisive. For example, poppy prices could reflect the results of expanding poppy production in recent years as much as fentanyl's entry into the market. But there are hints that fentanyl's rise might lead to less heroin being consumed, which also has been observed in Estonia, Canada, and Latvia to varying degrees.

Scenario 4: Coexisting Heroin and Synthetic Opioid Markets

In the previous scenario, we imagined that users were indifferent about whether their MEDs were natural or synthetic, but that might not be the case (see, e.g., Carroll et al., 2017; Ciccarone, Ondocsin, and Mars, 2017; BCCSU, 2019). If some users are willing to pay more per MED to get natural or semisynthetic rather than synthetic opioids, that raises the question of whether a heroin and a fentanyl market could coexist in North America, as opposed to fentanyl driving heroin out completely.

Coexistence is a real-world scenario; a form of it has already occurred in Sweden. However, in a famous paper, George Akerlof (1970) theorized that when a market contains lemons (or in this case, fentanyl, from the perspective of those who prefer heroin), no one will be willing to sell peaches (heroin) if users cannot figure out which product is which before purchase. That is, the presence of knockoff products might undermine the market for the legitimate product. Akerlof's example was low- and high-quality used cars, because the seller knows more about the quality of the car than the buyer does.

The lemons dynamic has always lurked in drug markets because cutting a bag of heroin with inert diluents does not change its appearance. Reuter and Caulkins (2004) and Galenianos, Pacula, and Persico (2012) analyzed this problem and concluded that drug markets might have survived the lemons problem in the past because of trust between dealers and users built up through repeated interaction.

However, fentanyl is a "sweeter lemon"; unlike diluents, it is a μ-opioid receptor agonist, just like heroin. Indeed, it is even more potent, and maybe some other, yet-to-be-marketed synthetic opioid will come even closer to matching heroin's unique "taste." A market equilibrium with higher-cost natural and semisynthetic opioids might be harder to maintain when the cheap imitation products close the quality gap.

Indeed, although Carroll et al. (2017, p. 140) describes users in Rhode Island who dislike fentanyl and actively seek to avoid it, "the avoidance of fentanyl-contaminated heroin was consistently described as difficult to impossible to achieve." Several users described "maintaining long-term relationships with trusted dealers" (Carroll et al., 2017, p. 143). McKnight and Des Jarlais (2018) also found users in New York City who tried to buy from the same dealer for this reason, but they report that few had such an arrangement. They found others who thought that this tactic was not very effective. One said, "You can know your dealer, but you [still] don't know what's in the bag."

These vignettes point to two possibilities. One is that the fentanyl-as-lemon problem pushes heroin distribution into transactions embedded within long-term stable relationships, and so alters—but does not collapse—the heroin market. Perhaps heroin-only sellers could provide fentanyl test strips so that users could certify that the bags offered as heroin in fact contain no fentanyl.[10]

The other possibility is that, even if some users would pay more for heroin, the market cannot coexist with a fentanyl market filled with people who shop based on "kick for the buck." In this case, heroin would be relegated to distinct niches where it does not compete head-to-head with fentanyl.

At present, it is fentanyl that is associated with internet-enabled e-commerce, and in Sweden, where heroin and fentanyl markets have coexisted, it is heroin that dominates traditional street markets. However, one could imagine the opposite situation, with fentanyl driving heroin out of street markets populated by low-income users who are price-sensitive, while leaving a crypto market that serves discerning heroin customers who want to be protected from fentanyl's risks. Indeed, Gilbert and Dasgupta (2017) describes cryptomarkets that prohibit the sale of fentanyl or carfentanil. Of course, adulteration also can happen in online cryptomarkets (Quintana et al., 2017; van der Gouwe et al., 2017). Still, the online user forums associated with cryptomarkets might be able to enforce norms more effectively than could users in traditional street markets (Karamouzian et al., 2018; Quintana et al., 2017).

A Corollary: Violence Prevention Through Chemistry?

If synthetic opioids drive heroin out of most markets, it could erode the power of the DTOs that dominate Mexico's poppy-growing areas and cut their revenues from cross-border smuggling operations (Humphreys, Caulkins, and Felbab-Brown, 2018). In the short run, this might generate more violence as the DTOs compete for a declining market, but in the long run, it could reduce violence and corruption in Mexico (Kilmer et al., 2010).

---

[10] Testing for the presence or absence of fentanyl is easier and cheaper than is quantitative testing to establish how much fentanyl a sample contains.

At the other end of the distribution chain, fentanyl could conceivably soften the long-standing association between individuals suffering from OUD and economic-compulsive crime. If fentanyl supplied MEDs cheaply enough to make retail prices fall (and that is an important and unresolved "if"), then those with OUD might have less need to commit economic-compulsive crime to finance their purchases. That higher opioid prices can lead to higher rates of acquisitive crime and vice versa has long been recognized. Indeed, in one of the first serious studies of the price responsiveness of heroin use, Silverman and Spruill (1977) found that, if heroin prices in Detroit went up by 50 percent, there would be a 14-percent increase in total property crime. However, the relationship could be complicated by how price changes affect income from drug dealing (Bretteville-Jensen and Sutton, 1996).[11]

There is an argument, admittedly more speculative, for why online distribution might reduce systemic drug-related violence in wholesale and retail markets. Heroin, cocaine, and methamphetamine are distributed to U.S. markets through multilevel chains dominated at every level by criminals with a capacity for violence, and transactions usually involve in-person meetings. One view holds that the ubiquitous capacity for violence is a necessary and structural consequence of product illegality; when disputes cannot be resolved in courts, negotiating parties might resort to force to resolve disagreements. However, neither heroin distribution in Europe nor cannabis distribution in North America are as closely associated with violence as are heroin markets in the United States or cannabis trafficking in Mexico. Thus, illegality might provide fertile fields for growing violence, but it might not plant the seed. Online distribution could reduce opportunities for in-person transactions that might result in violence and obviate the need for armed and potentially violent criminals to smuggle product across borders.

---

[11] Income from theft declined for the Oslo drug injectors studied by Bretteville-Jensen and Sutton over a period when prices were falling, but it is hard to know whether it was declining prices that caused the decline in property crime (personal communication with Bretteville-Jensen, April 8, 2019).

One (untested) hypothesis for why drug distribution in the United States is more violent than in Europe is that proclivity for violence at one level "infects" organizations at adjacent market levels with which there are direct interactions. Production and cross-border smuggling into the United States are dominated by Mexican DTOs that have an extreme capacity for violence. Perhaps the only people who would risk meeting with and buying from such violent criminals are other criminals with a capacity for violence. In turn, the customers of those organizations might also need some capacity to threaten and deliver violence to avoid being cheated themselves, and so on down the line.

If midlevel dealers can buy fentanyl over the internet from a distant supplier with whom they never meet face to face, it might eliminate the need for the midlevel dealer to be armed. Indeed, the key might not be that the deal is arranged online so much as that the drugs are delivered via mail or commercial package delivery, rather than being hand-delivered by the criminal supplier, and/or that payments are made in such cryptocurrencies as Bitcoin, rather than in cash (Gilbert and Dasgupta, 2017; Kruithof et al., 2016).[12]

Under this theory, there are at least three reasons why direct mail import of fentanyl could cut systemic violence. First, it eliminates several violent layers of the distribution chain. Second, because fentanyl can be imported by stealth, rather than by corruption or violence, the top of its distribution chain within U.S. borders might be less violent. Drug couriers might carry guns; FedEx couriers do not. Third, if lower-level dealers need to be tough in order to deal with tough suppliers, then making the top of the chain less violent might make the rest of the chain less violent as well.

There is an interesting parallel with the distribution of prescription opioids earlier in the opioid epidemic. Large-scale diversion from the wholesale supply chain was relatively rare (National Academies of Sciences, 2017); most of the diversion happened at the prescriber-patient level (e.g., by doctor shopping, medication pilfering, underregulated pain management clinics, etc.). As a result, there were relatively

---

[12] Of course, there also is a possibility of fentanyl being directly supplied to at least some users, thus bypassing local dealers.

few criminal kingpins in prescription opioid distribution; it was largely people with OUD and multiple prescriptions feeding their own habit, and maybe those of a few friends. This meant that distribution of prescription opioids was primarily a health problem (overdose and OUD), rather than a violence problem, such as the crack epidemic in the 1980s with its open-air drug markets and drive-by shootings.

The parallel is not that fentanyl will be diverted from medical use. That has always happened to a degree, but the modern fentanyl epidemic is primarily about purely illegal distribution (see Chapter One). However, if individuals with OUD could obtain drugs from online vendors that ship directly to their homes, fentanyl could spread with no more violence than oxycodone did in the early days of pill mills.

Of course, this is an exaggeration: Webpages selling 10 g of fentanyl are likely selling to low-level wholesale dealers, not directly to users. Still, we can imagine a world in which thousands of low-level dealers order supplies online, rather than meet with violent kingpins, and then distribute the drugs to friends, rather than via street markets. That would be a world in which no U.S. drug gang gets enormously rich and powerful or hires lookouts, touts, or men with guns.

Three Uncertainties That Might Influence Which Scenario Transpires

Cost considerations tend to point to fentanyl sweeping heroin aside, but three possibilities might moderate that spread, at least in some places.

Does it Take a Shortage to Trigger Substitution on the Supply Side?

In a theoretical market with no search costs, a lower-cost option will always drive out an equivalent higher-cost option, even when the cost difference is minor. But in the real world, people are reluctant to change. Some people stick with an electricity, cell phone, insurance, or cable provider even when a competitor offers essentially the same product for a lower price (Wilson and Price, 2010).

One might expect that drug dealers, as businesspeople, would quickly jump on opportunities to cut costs, even if consumers do not.

Yet, as Boyum (1992) observes, drug markets are different. They might be highly competitive in some respects, but there are no strong selection pressures favoring cost containment: Even a poorly managed drug distribution operation still produces positive cash flow.

This allows drug distribution groups to be quite conservative, in the sense of sticking with old ways of doing business until forced to adapt by a shortage. As we described in Chapter Four, one can tell Estonia's peculiar story with fentanyl through this lens. Those in Estonia used heroin until the Taliban's poppy ban created a shortage in 2001, and only in 2002 did Estonia become known for its fentanyl market after dealers adopted this substitute.

Mounteney et al. (2015) likewise describes fentanyl as having emerged in some places that were affected by heroin shortages, and Hempstead and Yildirim (2014) argues something similar for New Jersey at the time of the 2006 fentanyl outbreak. This school of thought also would observe that, although alpha-methylfentanyl appeared in California drug markets in 1979 (Henderson, 1988; Ojanpera et al., 2008), it did not become common until a large population that had become dependent on opioids was cut off from that supply.

If this story is true—and it might not be—then fentanyl could come to dominate in North America and yet not make inroads in Europe, as long as Europe continues to have a stable, uninterrupted supply of heroin from Afghanistan.

However, there are counterexamples to the idea that fentanyl needed a market disruption to gain a foothold. To the best of our knowledge, there is no claim of any heroin shortage in Canada preceding the spread of fentanyl there, although a stable supply might not have been able to meet an influx of demand from individuals who were looking for alternatives to prescription opioids. Nor is the evidence of a U.S. shortage really compelling, although that reflects, in part, the poor quality of data on price and purity.

So if fentanyl can only take hold when existing illegal opioid markets are disrupted, an absence of further such disruptions might limit the spread of fentanyl. However, at this point, it is not clear whether such disruptions are truly a necessary precondition.[13] Nor is it clear whether, in a place where heroin is rare but non-medical use of prescription opioids is common, there needs to be a disruption in the supply of prescription opioids for fentanyl to make inroads. Arguably, West Virginia was such a place, and it was hit hard by fentanyl even though it is not clear whether its prescription opioid market was disrupted around the time that fentanyl spread.

Do Users Like Synthetic Opioids as Much as Heroin?

All opioids are substitutes for each other to some degree, and MED conversion charts can lull one into thinking that the opioid agonists are indistinguishable, apart from variation in potency. But they are not.[14] For example, there is evidence that some people with OUD who have not responded to conventional treatment might respond better to heroin-assisted treatment (HAT) than to methadone (Demaret et al., 2015; Haasen et al., 2007; Kilmer et al., 2018; March et al., 2006; Strang et al., 2015).

This raises the question of whether users like fentanyl or its analogs enough for them to displace heroin when heroin continues to be available. As far as we know, the scientific literature does not provide a definitive answer. There are reports of individuals actively seeking out fentanyl (Vestal, 2019), but there are also reports that many more opioid users prefer heroin to fentanyl (80 percent versus 16 percent; BCCSU, 2019).

Based on a mixed-methods study of 149 opioid users in Rhode Island, Carroll and colleagues reports that those users "described fentanyl as unpleasant, potentially deadly, and to be avoided" and "reported limited ability to identify fentanyl in their drugs," although some thought that fentanyl could be detected by sight or smell (Carroll

---

[13] For example, one factor not associated with a shortage is the modus operandi contagion effect (i.e., organized crime groups and other nonstate actors learning from each other and copying each other's techniques). This effect, observed in the context of illicit economies and terrorism studies, would suggest that new criminal groups might start supplying fentanyl after learning about its advantages (see, e.g., Nesser and Stenersen, 2014).

[14] Even the simplistic view would recognize that partial agonists, such as buprenorphine and tramadol, are different.

et al., 2017, p. 136). Another telling quote is that "a general consensus emerged that the effects of fentanyl are distinctively uncomfortable or distressing" (Carroll, 2017, p. 140).

However, the next paper in the same journal reports different conclusions based on an ethnographic study of 38 heroin users in a neighboring state. Ciccarone and colleagues reports that "Respondents expressed a wide range of opinions on the type of 'heroin' they preferred. . . . Among proponents of perceived fentanyl, the powerful rush sensation . . . was always listed as among the principal benefits. . . . The primary negative quality of [fentanyl-adulterated or substituted heroin] was its short duration" (Ciccarone, Ondocsin, and Mars, 2017, p. 149). Users in that study also liked fentanyl's ability to overcome tolerance and opiate receptor–blocking medication and reported various signs that they believed helped them tell whether fentanyl was present. Firestone, Goldman, and Fischer (2009) reports that, in Toronto, diverted pharmaceutical fentanyl was highly desired and commanded a premium price.

Given these inconsistent reports from studies with individual users, it is also worth considering two case studies at the market level.

The first case study is Sweden, where fentanyl existed as a completely distinct market from heroin, not as a heroin adulterant (see Chapter Four). Fentanyl analogs were sold as such online with delivery by Swedish Post, usually in the form of nasal sprays. Heroin was sold in conventional street markets in major urban areas.

There are several hypotheses as to why there might be demand for fentanyl despite the existence of a stable heroin market, including availability in rural areas not well served by urban street markets, availability in forms that do not require injection, and the possibility that analogs would not be detected by drug tests. But the more pertinent question is why the street market for heroin persisted despite the availability of fentanyl. The answer might be something prosaic, such as lack of internet access and payment options, or the possibility that, absent some disruption to heroin supply, heroin users are content to continue using heroin.

The second case study is Baltimore, Maryland, as described by Mars, Ondocsin, and Ciccarone (2018a). Apparently, that city has two distinct opioid street markets—one for "raw" (thought to be traditional heroin without fentanyl) and the other for "scramble" (which is understood to be adulterated with fentanyl). Mars, Ondocsin, and Ciccarone (2018a) reports some geographic separation, with some neighborhoods traditionally having raw and others having scramble, and a price differential, with scramble considered to be cheaper. However, overall, these markets are much less separated than are the heroin and fentanyl markets in Sweden. In that sense, they are unlike anything seen in the international jurisdictions described in Chapter Four.

This evidence regarding user preference is inconclusive. It seems consistent with a belief that some people prefer heroin and others prefer fentanyl. However, it is also consistent with the idea that opioid users can get used to any opioid, whether heroin, fentanyl or, as in Finland, buprenorphine. If so, then whatever opioid has already been established (usually heroin) has an advantage over any challenger (often fentanyl). But this advantage is history-dependent, rather than intrinsic to the chemical compound.

Overall, the thinness of the scientific literature suggests a need for more research about which drug is preferred, under what conditions, and over what range of relative costs.

What if Fentanyl Is Not Much Cheaper for Users?

Fentanyl is much cheaper than heroin per MED at the import level (see Appendix B), but will that translate into lower prices for users? There is considerable literature discussing how changes in costs (or prices) far up the distribution chain do or do not percolate down to substantially alter retail prices (Caulkins, 2007). One view is that, because most of the increase in drug prices happens in the last few distribution layers, reductions in prices upstream are of little consequence for retail prices. If events transpired to make a drug that previously sold for $20 per gram at wholesale and $100 at retail now cost $40 per gram at wholesale, it might only push the retail price up to $120 per gram, rather than $200 (an additive, not a multiplicative, model of price transmission).

Indeed, although both the additive and multiplicative models would predict that retail prices should fall at least somewhat when wholesale prices fall, it is not clear that retail heroin prices as measured have actually fallen much in the years since fentanyl arrived. For that matter, although international price data are complicated, it is not clear that fentanyl's arrival drove retail opioid prices down elsewhere. The price per dose in Estonia's and Latvia's fentanyl markets is €10, and Latvia's heroin prices went up after fentanyl took away most of heroin's market share. Why have substantial declines in heroin prices not been observed yet in the United States?

One possibility is measurement error and bad data. Fentanyl is still mostly confined to the eastern United States, but heroin prices often are reported nationally. More fundamentally, fentanyl is an active ingredient, not a diluent. Adding fentanyl to a bag of heroin increases the number of MEDs in the bag, and the weight changes little because fentanyl is so potent. Thus, it would not be surprising if both the total price and price per gram of the mixed bag went up, even if the price per MED went down. Because heroin prices are quoted per pure gram of heroin, rather than per MED, it is possible that fentanyl has lowered the price per MED, even if heroin price series report no decline. That is, current methods of monitoring heroin prices might fail to account for the realities of street bags containing multiple opioids. Yet another complication is that users do not always know whether they are buying heroin, fentanyl, or a mixture of the two and sometimes use a generic term, such as "down" or "dope" for opioids generally.

It also is possible that heroin prices will drop significantly later because, as Kleiman (1989) observes, prices are set by the marginal producer. Even if other, "inframarginal" producers' cost structures are much lower, retail price will stay high until those inframarginal producers can meet all demand and higher-cost producers are driven out of the market. The fentanyl supply chain might not yet move sufficient volumes to meet all demand for illegal opioids.

That situation should not last indefinitely in a competitive market with free entry, but perhaps the five years since fentanyl's arrival is not a very long time in the context of drug markets, with their slow information flows. After all, it seems to have taken most of the 1980s for cocaine to drop to prices that were justified by the costs of distribution (Caulkins and Reuter, 1996).

In summary, fentanyl's compelling advantages from the perspective of drug traffickers suggest that—to the extent that anything is predictable about drug markets—it is a relatively safe bet that synthetic opioids will persist where they have become established and over time will expand to displace heroin, at least to a degree. However, a preference for the familiar on the part of those who use drugs, as well as by some dealers, could moderate the speed of that spread.

CHAPTER SIX

Concluding Thoughts

Fentanyl and other synthetic opioids in the illicit market kill on an unprecedented scale. As we discussed in the preceding chapters, the causes, dynamics, and future course of fentanyl and synthetic opioid use are fundamentally different from those of other modern drug epidemics. These differences are not widely appreciated, and they matter for how policymakers and society more broadly respond. The differences do not imply that standard approaches to reducing substance use disorders and poisonings should be abandoned (e.g., increasing treatment, reducing supply). Those strategies remain important, but they are not enough.

Synthesizing information from the previous chapters, we identify five key insights about fentanyl and synthetic opioids that are integral to any complete, empirically grounded understanding of this problem. We then consider what those insights imply for the strengths and limitations of the four traditional and complementary pillars of drug policy (supply control, prevention, treatment, and harm reduction). We conclude by presenting some policy options that might deserve discussion and analysis. The inadequacy of the usual approaches, given the realities of the synthetic opioid environment, implies that other options should be on the table.

In Appendix C, we offer a technical adjunct, most of which focuses on efforts to improve data collection and surveillance specific to this growing problem. While the United States has been experiencing unprecedented increases in overdoses, the nation's data infrastructure for monitoring and understanding drug problems has been crumbling.

It was never particularly well-suited to monitoring synthetic opioids or other novel psychoactives, and neglect has diminished its ability to track both market supply and the pool of people suffering from OUD. Appendix C offers ideas for improving surveillance and monitoring to better address the synthetic opioid problem.

Five Basic Insights About the Challenge of Synthetic Opioids

We discuss five basic insights about synthetic opioids that should be borne in mind when discussing policy responses to this issue.

Problems with Synthetic Opioids Are Likely to Worsen Before They Improve, and States West of the Mississippi River Must Remain Vigilant

One of the most important—and depressing—insights from the preceding analysis is that, however bad the synthetic opioid problem is now, it is likely to get worse before it gets better. In Chapter Two, we showed that the nation's synthetic opioid problem is not yet truly national in scope. Some regions have been acutely affected; others have been spared to date, at least in relative terms, but they should not be complacent.

The math is simple and distressing. If the entire nation had a death rate of even half of what New England experienced in 2017, it would imply a substantial increase in deaths. Potent synthetic opioids appearing in counterfeit prescription medications is another concern. Those using diverted prescription pain relievers or other medications could be at substantial risk of overdose, should they assume that these fakes are of genuine origin.

The problem could worsen in other ways. Currently, synthetic opioids appear in the postmortems of about half of overdose deaths involving cocaine and about one-quarter of overdoses involving psychostimulants (mostly methamphetamine), again with sharp regional variation. For example, in Ohio, about seven out of ten cocaine overdoses involve synthetic opioids. Some users knowingly ingested heroin along with cocaine (sometimes referred to as *speedballing*) or meth-amphetamine (sometimes referred to as *goofballing*). Such trends are worrisome because stimulant-only users are not opioid-tolerant and are much more likely to overdose if they simultaneously use opioids, especially fentanyl. Although some might mix these drugs for pleasure, there is anecdotal evidence that some individuals are mixing in stimulants to counteract the sedating effects of fentanyl (Szalavitz, 2019). Others ingested stimulants that already contained fentanyl, although it is not clear whether dealers intentionally adulterate stimulants with fentanyl or if it is accidental cross-contamination (Daly, 2019). Either way, if cocaine users on the West Coast or more methamphetamine users generally become exposed to synthetic opioids, death rates would increase. In 2019, authorities reported multiple overdoses in California after individuals consumed fentanyl thought to be cocaine (Armenian et al., 2019; Byik, 2019).

Furthermore, fentanyl is not the most potent synthetic opioid. As noted in Chapter Two, in 2017, Ohio and British Columbia saw surges in deaths associated with carfentanil. Carfentanil was, until recently, the clearly dominant synthetic opioid in Latvia (see Chapter Four).

In Chapter Five, we offered multiple scenarios for the future trajectories of fentanyl and other synthetic opioids in the United States and the factors that could shape them. No one knows how the trajectories will actually evolve, but it would be prudent to prepare for the problem to get worse before it gets better and to anticipate that it will persist for the indefinite future, rather than flash and recede.

Supplier Decisions, Not User Demand, Drive the Transition to Fentanyl

The history of drug use and drug problems in the United States has been characterized by a sequence of "epidemics," but the synthetic opioid problem is different. Whereas previous epidemics in contemporary North America were fueled by growing demand, this one appears to be supply-driven. To date, it primarily involves an adulterant, rather than the drug that most users seek out by name.[1] Thus, fentanyl is best thought of as a strategic device for dealers seeking to lower costs rather than a newly popular drug among users.

To elaborate, historically, most drug epidemics begin with rapid, even contagious spread of initiation, primarily among youth and often amid ignorance, overconfidence, or naivete about the drug's risks. Over time, as some users escalate to frequent and/or chronic use, the reputation of the drug changes. Then initiation ebbs, and society is left to deal with a residual pool of chronic users whose use persists, often for decades (Courtwright, 2009; Musto, 1999).

Almost none of that script pertains to fentanyl. Fentanyl use typically does not spread by word-of-mouth contact among users; it penetrates markets when suppliers embrace it. Very few opioid users who were not previously exposed to fentanyl are looking for it or other synthetic opioids; indeed, many longtime heroin users prefer not to use these substances, given their lethality and unpredictability, although some come to prefer fentanyl because of its ability to overcome tolerance (Ciccarone, Ondocsin, and Mars, 2017; Mars, Ondocsin, and Ciccarone, 2018b). Given these facts, the traditional epidemic framework fails to capture the dynamics of the problem.

Synthetic Opioids Drive Up Deaths Rather Than the Number of Users

In Chapter Four, we observed that injection drug use in Estonia peaked in the 1990s, before the arrival of fentanyl. Elsewhere in Europe, the emergence of fentanyl generally occurred against the backdrop of declining opioid user populations. Likewise, we have not come across evidence pointing to fentanyl increasing either initiation or chronic use in the United States or Canada (although household surveys do not ask about fentanyl initiation). Although OUD is far more common than it was 20 years ago, that growth primarily came from prescription opioids and happened before 2014, not from fentanyl in the past few years.

---

[1] It is possible that, over time, fentanyl will become not only the dominant opioid but also the preferred opioid, especially in users with high tolerance. "Good is what you are used to" (personal communication with F. H. Reuter). Interviewees commenting on Estonia felt that after 15 years, opioid users in that country will have no interest in returning to heroin.

Hence, it seems fair to say that fentanyl triggered a wave of deaths and not a rising tide of more users.

That this problem is so different suggests that the response will also need to be different. Although traditional approaches aimed at drug epidemics focus on preventing initiation, raising prices, and increasing treatment to suppress demand, these efforts will not immediately reduce overdose deaths in areas that are already awash in synthetic opioids. Reducing deaths quickly will require consideration of interventions intended to reduce the risk of drug overdose or exposure to potent synthetic opioids that are still controversial in the United States (see, e.g., McGinty et al., 2018; Kilmer et al., 2019).

A focus on reducing deaths and nonfatal synthetic opioid poisonings does not mean that jurisdictions should abandon traditional approaches to reducing consumption and OUD. Fentanyl has driven death rates up sharply in multiple countries that pursue diverse policies. It is clear that some nontraditional, outside-the-box thinking will be required to address this new challenge.

Fentanyl's Spread Is Episodically Fast and Has Ratchet-Like Persistence

If one asks whether fentanyl spreads quickly or slowly, the best answer appears to be "yes." Once dealers begin to substitute fentanyl for heroin, it might be only a short time before the drug is capable of sweeping through a market. In Chapter Two, we described how, in just a few years, fentanyl practically drove heroin out of many markets in New Hampshire. That said, in Chapter Two, we also noted that death rates from synthetic opioids remain far lower in a large swath of the western United States than the rates in New England. Illegally manufactured fentanyl is not totally absent from the west, but it remains a minor presence.[2]

One possible explanation for these seemingly contradictory observations is that some illegal markets appear to require a certain mini-

---

[2] Heroin in the western United States is mostly Mexican "black tar" heroin, and some believe that it is physically difficult to mix fentanyl into that type of heroin. If so, we should not be surprised if some inventive chemists make it a goal to find easier ways to adulterate black tar heroin with fentanyl or produce a tar variant containing fentanyl but no heroin.

mum scale to operate efficiently. Below that scale, an illegal market struggles. Above that scale, the market is resilient to enforcement and other disruptions. Such a situation can lead two otherwise similar places to have very different rates of use, low in one market and high in another, and for those different states to be stable over time.

It appears that fentanyl can be slow to make inroads, particularly in the face of competition from heroin or other opioids, but once it has entered the market, it can expand rapidly and even drive out other opioids.

This "tipping" from a low- to a high-volume equilibrium of fentanyl sales appears to be a one-way ratchet. Although multiple minor fentanyl outbreaks in the United States and abroad have fizzled (see Chapters Three and Four), there are no instances we could find in which a substantial market with an established synthetic opioid supply has reverted to heroin.

One could crudely divide the world into two types of areas: those already beset by fentanyl and those that are fighting to delay their transition. The second group has reason to be vigilant. Although prompt action could extinguish nascent fires, as happened, for example, in the United States from 2005 to 2007, the window of opportunity is small and might be closing. Prior outbreaks were attributable to a single supply source. The arrival of mass-produced and cheap imports is no longer tied to a single source.

The Internet Revolution in Drug Trafficking

Daniel Wilson wrote an entertaining parody of overly optimistic futurist scenarios entitled *Where's My Jetpack?: A Guide to the Amazing Science Fiction Future That Never Arrived* (Wilson, 2018). If he had been a student of drug policy, he might have included a chapter on how the dark web and cryptocurrencies would revolutionize drug trafficking, leading to widespread layoffs in traditional DTOs. Academics have been writing about the illegal distribution of opioids over the internet for more than a decade (Forman, 2003) and about the dark web's potential for disrupting drug distribution more generally for quite some time (e.g., Aldridge and Décary-Hétu, 2014; Barratt, 2012). However, well into the age of the internet, cryptomarket drug sales appeared to be in the hundreds of millions of dollars per year (Kruithof et al., 2016), whereas overall retail drug sales in the United States were more than $100 billion (Midgette et al., 2019). Thus, it is with some trepidation that we observe that fentanyl distribution has established a precedent for a fundamental shift in the nature of drug distribution. In Chapter Five, we outlined the basic argument: Internet-enabled sales and direct distribution by mail or package delivery to low- or midlevel wholesale dealers can be a much cheaper way to distribute drugs than traditional distribution networks.

Although fentanyl is unusually compact because it is so potent, similar considerations apply to other drugs. In round terms, the price of 1 kg of cocaine rises from about $5,000 in South or Central America to about $15,000 or more in U.S. wholesale markets. In a sense, DTOs "charge" $10,000 per kilogram to ship cocaine into the country. However, as noted in Chapter Three, private consignment carriers will ship a 1-kg package from China to the United States for closer to $100, or about 1 percent as much (or one-tenth that amount via international post).

Expressing this in terms of shipping cost per dose is also instructive. If a dose of fentanyl weighs a few milligrams, then mailing costs of $100 per kilogram shrink below a tenth of a penny per dose. Parallel arithmetic for a 100-mg dose of cocaine still points to shipping costs of only a penny for doses that now sell for more than $10 on the street. Whether shipping costs are a fraction of a penny or a full penny per dose is probably of little consequence.

Of course, the full cost of shipping drugs needs to include a premium to compensate for the risks of arrest, violence, and drug seizures. However, the first two risks are conspicuously low for an overseas organization operating in territory that is fairly immune to the pressures of U.S. law enforcement, and there are multiple such havens.

All of this suggests that the internet could upend the distribution of many drugs, not just fentanyl. A Wild West of unregulated online drug bazaars sounds like a public health nightmare, but it would be a Wild West without gunfights, or at least with fewer than occur today. Therefore, this revolution—if it ever comes—could, like many technological revolutions, have both favorable and unfavorable effects. In any

event, policymakers designing drug strategies might wish to consider the possibility that over the next 20 years, the internet could disrupt drug distribution networks generally.[3]

Rethinking Drug Policy in the Context of Synthetic Opioids

Drug policy is typically divided into four pillars (supply control, prevention, treatment, and harm reduction), and discussions of the relative merits of these pillars occupies a central place in drug policy debates. The synthetic opioid crisis, however, deeply challenges all of the traditional approaches (see Box 1).

Fentanyl's challenge to supply control. Because supply control's main contribution has been to keep prices high, and because fentanyl cuts the wholesale price per MED by roughly 99 percent, the time may be coming when the United States can no longer think of high prices as the first line of defense against wider use of opioids. Indeed, increasing the price of heroin through better supply control might increase the attractiveness of fentanyl for dealers (Mars, Rosenblum, and Ciccarone, 2018). However, as we discussed, there are good arguments for trying to reduce or prevent fentanyl supply in order to buy time, particularly in parts of the country where synthetic opioids are not yet common.

Fentanyl's challenge to conventional prevention. Fentanyl is spreading primarily because suppliers are cutting costs, not because users are asking for fentanyl. Indeed, many of fentanyl's victims did not want or even know that they were using it. Furthermore, expanding school-based prevention, a major focus of conventional preven-

---

[3]   Consider a scenario in which international exporters supply low-level wholesale dealers through one or two intermediaries, rather than the five or more layers common in contemporary drug distribution networks.

Box 1. Opioids and the Traditional Drug Policy Pillars

The first pillar is *supply control*, ranging from poppy eradication and substitution to interdiction and domestic law enforcement against drug dealers or those who improperly dispense prescription medications. U.S. drug policy for decades was heavily focused, both in budgetary and substantive terms, on supply-reduction efforts (Kleiman, 2009). Collectively, these expensive efforts keep prices high (the common drugs sell for much more than their weight in gold), but they rarely create physical scarcity. High prices are a mixed blessing. They can hold down substance use disorders, but they also enrich dealers while impoverishing those with substance use disorders, some of whom commit crimes to finance drug purchases (Gallett, 2014).

The second pillar, *prevention*, is broadly esteemed despite its mediocre performance when evaluated rigorously (Babor et al., 2018). If you give 100 youths who would otherwise have used drugs the best available prevention programming, most will still go on to use drugs. Altering the paths of the minority who do respond can well justify the investment. However, even the effectiveness of model programs does not approach that of vaccinations for measles or other childhood diseases (Strang et al., 2012).

The third pillar, *treatment* for those who have developed an OUD, has the strongest evidence base, particularly for methadone and other forms of medication treatment. Medication treatment can stabilize people's lives; reduce cravings associated with addiction, reduce overdose and the spread of HIV and other infectious diseases; and facilitate access to other social services (Mattick et al., 2009; Mattick et al., 2014; McLellan et al., 1993; McLellan et al., 1998). It is also a long-term endeavor and is often punctuated by recurrence of street drug use. It is not something

---

Box 1—Continued

with a dependably favorable short-term outcome, such as setting a broken arm. Furthermore, many who meet the medical definition of "needing" treatment do not seek it, some who want it cannot find it, and many who begin treatment drop out.

Recognizing the inevitability of continued use by some of those who enter treatment by those who do not want or cannot access treatment, many developed countries also embrace *harm-reduction* programs that make continued use safer and less damaging to people who use drugs and those around them. The main harm-reduction programs in the United States include distributing sterile syringes to those who inject drugs, administering naloxone after someone overdoses, and training people who use drugs and other members of the community to carry and administer naloxone.

---

tion efforts, will do little to directly reduce today's appalling death toll among people in their 30s and 40s.[4]

Fentanyl's challenge to treatment. A quick look at the numbers suggests that the country probably will not be able to treat its way out of the fentanyl problem. Even in Western Europe, where treatment is generally better funded and more readily available, the annual non-AIDS mortality rate of individuals who inject drugs was already 1.4 deaths per 100 person-years before the arrival of fentanyl (Mathers and Degenhardt, 2014). An important subset of those deaths came from overdose. The risk of death is about 70-percent lower during

---

[4]   There may well be a role for educating existing users about safer ways to use. Just as Mothers Against Drunk Driving altered norms surrounding alcohol use ("friends don't let friends drive drunk"), one could imagine altering norms about the use of street drugs ("friends don't let friends use opioids alone"). Such efforts, however, are more in the spirit of harm reduction than traditional drug prevention. Some of these messaging campaigns are currently under way (see, e.g., the DOPE Project, a San Francisco–based harm reduction initiative; Harm Reduction Coalition, [undated]).

medication treatment (Mathers and Degenhardt, 2014), but the risk is not zero and those who inject drugs often cycle in and out of medication treatment.

If fentanyl's penetration of opioid markets increases the non-AIDS death rate markedly, as it almost certainly does, then the cumulative death risk can become substantial over time, even for people who have access to treatment. Specific numbers are not known, but suppose for the sake of illustration that, in the era of fentanyl, the all-cause death rate for those who inject drugs increases to 3 percent per year outside of treatment, with medication cutting that by 70 percent. The chance of surviving for 15 years with half of those years spent in treatment and half using street drugs would only be three in four. That would put the survival rate of OUD slightly above that of kidney or colon cancer and well below that of breast cancer (Jemal et al., 2010). The idea that something like one in four people with OUD who use street drugs might eventually die as a result, even if they have access to medication therapy is sobering, given estimates that there might be more than 3 million people with OUD in the United States.[5]

That said, expanding access to available treatment options and considering other innovative treatment modalities is paramount to reducing exposure to fentanyl. Overdose deaths would be higher without medication therapies; still, policymakers should not place all their hopes on treatment (or prevention, for that matter) as the sole solution to this problem. More information is needed to optimize treatment availability and deployment when facing fentanyl's potency and unpredictability in illicit markets.

---

[5] Based on the National Survey on Drugs and Health (NSDUH), Center for Behavioral Health Statistics and Quality (2017) estimates that 2.1 million people ages 12 or older had an OUD in 2016; however, NSDUH is notorious for missing those who use heroin on a daily or near daily (DND) basis. Caulkins et al. (2015) shows that, in 2010, when there were probably close to 1 million DND heroin users, NSDUH estimated that there were only about 60,000, or 6 percent as many. Estimates of DND heroin users for 2016 were on the order of 1.5 million (Midgette et al., 2019). If 75 percent of the 1.5 million DND heroin users suffer from OUD (a likely conservative estimate), that would suggest that the number of individuals ages 12 and older with an OUD in 2016 was closer to 3 million (2.1 million + 1.5 million × [1–6 percent] × 0.75 = 3.16 million).

Fentanyl's challenge to harm reduction. Harm reduction is more controversial in the United States than in many developed countries; thus, the country does not have many programs or much variety. For example, some estimates suggest that there are fewer than 400 syringe service programs (SSPs) operating nationwide (North American Syringe Exchange Network, undated). Although sterile injecting equipment can reduce the spread of disease and infection, by itself it does not do much to reduce overdoses.[6]

It is not just the rather anemic harm reduction efforts in the United States that cannot cope with fentanyl. Fentanyl's challenge to treatment and harm reduction is etched starkly in Vancouver's death rate. Few cities have embraced treatment and harm reduction more energetically than Vancouver. Before fentanyl, that seemed to have worked well; HIV/AIDS was contained and heroin overdose death rates in British Columbia fell from an average of eight per 100,000 people from 1993 to 1999 to five per 100,000 from 2000 to 2012 (British Columbia Coroners Service, 2019). However, those policies, programs, and services have been challenged by fentanyl. British Columbia now has one of the highest opioid-related death rates (more than 30 per 100,000 in 2017 and 2018), which is higher than that in all but five U.S. jurisdictions.[7] The rate in Vancouver's health service delivery area is even higher (55 per 100,000 people).

These death rates are high, not only relative to opioid overdose deaths elsewhere but also in absolute terms. It is hard for many people who are not epidemiologists to understand whether death rates of 30 or 55 per 100,000 are large or small, so it might be useful to contrast them with death rates in the United States from homicide (4.8 per

---

[6] One could argue that SSPs make it easier for PWID to ask for and receive help when they need it. If this leads to an increase in treatment utilization and/or other services (e.g., access to a shelter where they could be monitored), this could indirectly reduce the risk of overdose. Furthermore, many SSPs offer training in naloxone administration or other overdose mitigation techniques, such as using "tester" shots of smaller doses.

[7] Fentanyl was reported in 82 percent and 88 percent of accidental opioid deaths in British Columbia in 2017 and 2018, respectively (Special Advisory Committee on the Epidemic of Opioid Overdoses, 2019).

100,000) and traffic crashes (12.3 per 100,000), which are familiar, widely discussed, and often pertain to premature deaths of people.

Of course, those harm-reduction policies could be saving many lives. Presumably, death rates would be higher if not for those efforts (see, e.g., Irvine et al., 2019). However, the current approach fails to cope with fentanyl or heroin in absolute terms.

This sober assessment of current strategies does not suggest an about-face. Rather, the severity of the problem suggests continuing all of the traditional strategies, while looking for new ones. Over the long term, it is important to acknowledge that a new era could be coming when synthetic opioids are so cheap and ubiquitous that supply control will become less cost-effective.

Falling prices and a pivot to treatment and harm reduction need not be an unhappy scenario for law enforcement. Freeing law enforcement of the obligation to squelch supply across the board could allow it to focus on the most-noxious dealers and organizations and strive to minimize violence and corruption per kilogram delivered, rather than the number of kilograms supplied (Caulkins and Reuter, 2009; Greenfield and Paoli, 2012). In a way, this would let law enforcement focus on public safety, rather than an addiction prevention mission. Also, as noted in Chapter Five, falling prices might reduce the amount of economic-compulsive crime committed as a means to finance drug purchase.

Furthermore, even if supply control becomes less important in the long term, now is not a time to pull back. The benefits of supply and demand reduction can depend on the current stage of a particular drug epidemic (Caulkins, 2005; Tragler, Caulkins, and Feichtinger, 2001). Supply control could be more effective at preventing or delaying a substance from entering the market than at suppressing an established market. For example, shielding western states from fentanyl until better drug testing technology becomes available might save lives.

Just as there are many types of treatment, there also are many interventions intended to reduce supply, each of which comes with its own costs and benefits. Productive policy discussions about synthetic opioids will likely focus less on the pillars and more on specific interventions within those pillars. And, as noted in the next section, these conversations should not be limited to available interventions most often employed in the United States.

Novel Approaches Deserve Discussion and Analysis

The earlier discussion is not hopeful. The basic message is that the fentanyl problem is different and very bad, could get worse before it gets better, and renders existing strategies inadequate. That raises the question of what should be done.

There is near-universal support from expert bodies and government agencies for increasing access to medication treatment for OUD (e.g., Christie et al., 2017; National Academies of Sciences, 2017). We agree. That was the expert consensus before the arrival of synthetic opioids, and their proliferation makes the benefits of treatment all the greater because the costs of untreated OUD have become much higher.

However, knowing that treatment should be expanded should not be conflated with knowing how to solve the problem. As discussed, expanding treatment and other health and social services, even to levels attained in European countries or Canada, would not be enough because treatment alone might not reduce death rates to precrisis levels in areas swamped in synthetic opioids. Furthermore, treatment does not quickly shrink the pool of chronic users, and the usual trajectory of recovery via treatment involves multiple rounds of recurrent use. This is a cycle that fentanyl makes even more dangerous, especially because those whose use recurs after entering treatment are often more prone to overdosing after opioid tolerance subsides. (Sordo et al., 2017).

Some have argued for a truly massive treatment expansion, on the order of $100 billion over ten years (see Lopez, 2019).[8] There is no doubt that an expansion would help reduce the morbidity and mortality associated with OUD and other substance use disorders significantly in the long run.

---

[8] This expansion could include initiating treatment in more settings; sustaining treatment in high-risk populations, such as those who are justice-involved; and supporting more-robust and more-extensive treatment systems, such as hub and spoke models.

We suggest that, in addition to expanding conventional approaches, it might be time to invent new approaches and be open to trying ideas that seemed too risky or too alien in the past. After all, there is no physical law affirming that overdose deaths or other harms need move in strict proportion to the amount of drug use. This is demonstrated by the fact that, over the past six years, heroin-related deaths have apparently risen much more than have the number of heroin users (Hedegaard, Miniño, and Warner, 2018; Midgette et al., 2019). Conversely, one way to reduce future deaths and other consequences of OUD would be to reduce the number of deaths or other consequences per million use sessions or per million days of use.

In this section, we offer some ideas that are not part of the usual short list of policy options in the United States, but which illustrate the idea that there are opportunities to be innovative. This is in no way a comprehensive list, but we do seek breadth, and we mention options related to supply, treatment, and harm reduction to demonstrate that there are opportunities for innovation generally, not just in one pillar over another.

To be clear, we are not endorsing these options. The goal of this section is not to make specific policy recommendations or systematically assess costs and benefits, especially because the consequences of—and trade-offs associated with—these policies would likely differ depending on the attributes of the jurisdiction in question. Some of these options have not been tried, let alone studied systematically. Rather, what we advocate is serious consideration of a broad array of approaches considered nontraditional in the United States, rather than searching more narrowly among the usual list of programs, and we attempt to demonstrate the existence of such innovative ideas through examples.

Reconsidering the Dangers of Diverted OUD Treatment Medications

As noted earlier, the proliferation of synthetic opioids makes increasing access to medication treatments even more valuable. Both buprenorphine and methadone are heavily regulated in the United States. Such regulations have multiple motives, but a central concern has been fear that these substances will be diverted to the illicit market. If preventing

the diversion of methadone and buprenorphine would starve the illicit opioid market or limit it to heroin, such concerns might make sense. But in places that are already swamped with fentanyl and other synthetic opioids, it seems worth asking whether diversion of these medications is equally troubling. That is, fentanyl's spread both increases the need for freer access to methadone and buprenorphine while reducing a traditional concern regarding freer access.

The regulatory barriers are especially significant for methadone. Unlike in other countries, such as Canada, which recently allowed any doctor to prescribe methadone to those with OUD (Health Canada, 2018), methadone for OUD therapy can be obtained in the United States only from the specialty treatment sector. Furthermore, only one take-home dose per week is allowed during the first three months of treatment; all other doses are supervised. The number of permitted take-home doses rises slowly to two during the second three months of treatment and three during the third three months of treatment. Furthermore, those liberties are available only to individuals deemed responsible in handling unsupervised opioids; many people must go to the clinic every day to take their medication under supervision (SAMHSA, 2015). Concerns about diversion are illustrated elsewhere. In 2007, the DEA issued a moratorium on licensing mobile medical units that distribute methadone over concerns of potential diversion (Vestal, 2018).

Much remains to be studied about the likely consequences of relaxing restrictions on methadone and buprenorphine, but some decisionmakers are not waiting. For example, a police chief in Vermont announced that he would direct his department to no longer arrest those who were distributing buprenorphine on the illicit market. In March 2019, the Vermont Judiciary Committee passed a law to decriminalize the possession of buprenorphine without a prescription ("Committee Approves Bill Decriminalizing Drug," 2019).[9] Vancouver

---

[9]   Some suggest considering decriminalization more broadly, not just for buprenorphine. In 2017, the United Nations and WHO released a statement recommending the review and repeal of "laws that criminalize or otherwise prohibit . . . drug use or possession of drugs for personal use" (WHO, 2017). More recently, the United Nations System Chief Executives Board (2019) stated its commitment to "promote alternatives to conviction and punish-

has gone further, starting a pilot program to prescribe 50 opioid-using patients free access to hydromorphone (Dilaudid) pills that they can crush and inject at a supervised consumption site.[10]

Learning from Portugal

In the 1990s, Portuguese policymakers faced a public health emergency in the form of high rates of HIV transmission via injection drug use, mostly of heroin. A government-appointed commission developed 12 guidelines that became the basis of a new national drug strategy that stressed humanism, pragmatism, and participation (EMCDDA, 2011). One guideline was decriminalization of drug possession for personal use, and this Portuguese innovation is sometimes simplistically described as decriminalization (and is sometimes confused with legalization). Drug use is still prohibited, but it is not criminally sanctioned.

The new strategy robustly funded an innovative system of "dissuasion commissions," known as CDTs, that are operated by the Portuguese Ministry of Health and sited alongside other interventions, including treatment programs, homeless shelters, mobile disease prevention centers, and SSPs.[11]

When an individual is found to possess up to ten doses of any drug without evidence indicating participation in sales or supply, the drugs are seized and the case is transferred to the nearest CDT. The three-member commission meets with the individual to assess their

---

ment in appropriate cases, including the decriminalization of drug possession for personal use." Because some voters could see decriminalization on the ballot sooner rather than later (Kilmer and MacCoun, 2017), it might be time to start thinking about its potential consequences—both pro and con.

[10] Baker (2019) notes more about this pilot program: "According to Coco Culbertson, who is overseeing the program for PHS [a Vancouver-based nonprofit providing services to vulnerable groups], the dosage will be prescribed by a physician, and participants will be able to get up to five doses per day, to be injected under the supervision of PHS staff and volunteers. Culbertson said the pills, which are worth about 36 cents when bought legally, cost drug users $20–$30 on the street."

[11] The strategy also recommended establishing supervised consumption sites, although none were opened (EMCDDA, 2011).

drug-taking habits and determines the most appropriate course of action.

Most interventions involve cannabis, rather than opioids, and result in provisional suspension of the sentence. Fifteen percent involve referral to treatment, and 14 percent involve punitive ruling, such as warnings, fines, banning from certain places or from meeting certain people, obligation to attend drug education classes, and removal of professional or firearms licenses (EMCDDA, 2011). The law does not stipulate the additional sanctions that can be imposed on those who do not comply (Laqueur, 2015), and it is generally understood that those who are referred to treatment but do not enter are not sanctioned for noncompliance.

The suite of innovations appears to have produced favorable results. HIV transmission rates and drug-induced deaths declined, and self-reported use did not change substantially (Hughes and Stevens, 2010; Laqueur, 2015), but it is hard to parse out what caused what. As Hughes and Stevens (2010) notes, that policy change coincided with increased funding for drug treatment and outreach services; also, the demand for heroin was falling elsewhere in Europe.

To a degree, decriminalization only formalized what was already happening. In most cases, prosecutors were already waiving sanctions for possession of small amounts of drugs; very few users were convicted or serving time for drug possession even before decriminalization (Laqueur, 2015). Yet, Laqueur (2015) notes that arrests for possession fell and were replaced with citations. Decriminalization might have been necessary to allow CDTs and other social services to operate legally and with greater reach within an administrative environment.

In sum, the Portuguese example is an interesting case of a dramatic innovation in response to a public health crisis brought on by heroin that might serve as an inspiration, if not a template, for parallel innovation in the United States.

Piloting Novel, Evidence-Informed Treatment Modalities

Increasing the number of people receiving medication treatment is imperative, and perhaps expanding the number of approved medications would be of additional help. These additional medications might be especially useful in places where fentanyl is entrenched.

Prescribing heroin for OUD is prohibited under U.S. federal law, but it is done in Canada and some European countries (Kilmer et al., 2018). This approach, sometimes referred to as heroin-assisted treatment, or HAT, seeks to reduce patients' use of illicit heroin and help stabilize their lives.

HAT is very different from legalizing heroin, and it is not a first-line treatment, even in countries where it is available. HAT patients typically inject pharmaceutical-grade heroin two to three times per day under clinical supervision. In general, these patients have been using heroin for several years and have tried other treatments—such as methadone—multiple times but continue to consume illicit heroin.

Evidence from multiple randomized controlled trials indicates that supervised injectable HAT—with optional oral methadone—can offer benefits over oral methadone alone for treating OUD in some of these individuals (Ferri, Davoli, and Perucci, 2011; Smart, 2018; Strang et al., 2015). A review by Smart (2018) found strong evidence that HAT reduced the use of illicit heroin and suggestive evidence that it decreased criminal activity and improved some health outcomes.[12] The reductions in the use of street-sourced heroin by those receiving HAT is worth noting. While in treatment, these individuals might be less likely than those receiving only methadone to be exposed to fentanyl.

Although it is currently illegal to prescribe heroin in the United States, it would be legal to conduct medically supervised randomized controlled trials of HAT. Kilmer et al. (2018) and Pardo and Reuter (2018) argue that pilot randomized controlled trials should be conducted in the United States to assess the costs and benefits of HAT and

---

[12] According to Kilmer et al.'s (2018) summary of Smart (2018):

> In our review of the comparative effectiveness of HAT for patient-level outcomes, we consider the evidence base as showing strong support if all or almost all studies assessed comparative effectiveness for a given outcome, studies of comparable methodological quality did not find significant effects in opposing directions, and more than two-thirds of the relevant studies found significant effects in the same direction. If this third factor did not hold but statistically insignificant findings generally supported the same direction of the effect, we consider the evidence as suggestive (p. viii).

consider whether it makes sense to change federal law to expand this treatment option.

Other opioid agonist therapies could be piloted. For example, hydromorphone (trade name Dilaudid) has been piloted in Canada as an alternative opioid agonist therapy. There are only two randomized controlled trials on hydromorphone. Findings are promising, suggesting that outcomes are no different from HAT in treating long-term OUD (Oviedo-Joekes et al., 2016; Oviedo-Joekes et al., 2010). There also have been some studies suggesting that extended-release morphine could be beneficial for some OUD patients (Wells and Jones, 2017).[13]

Increasing Access to Drug Content Testing Technologies

If users had a cheap and easy way to test their drugs to see if those drugs contain fentanyl, then they might discard contaminated bags, or at least use them more cautiously.[14] By that logic, subsidizing distribution of a detection technology (for example, test strips that identify the presence of fentanyl in a bag of powder) might alter users' behaviors in ways that mitigate risks (Krieger et al., 2018; Peiper et al., 2019).

However, there are challenges with current technologies. Some tests are better at detecting metabolites than the original chemical, and so are better suited to testing urine for past use, rather than drug samples before use. Some tests might detect fentanyl, but not the newer analogs. Furthermore, if fentanyl completely replaces heroin in a market, then the relevant question is not whether a bag contains fen-

---

[13] Apart from these evidence-based therapies that seek to replace more-harmful and unregulated opioids with pharmaceutical-grade alternatives administered under medical supervision, there are some promising pharmacotherapies that have not undergone rigorous analysis. The best known is ibogaine, a psychoactive alkaloid found in the iboga plant. Its use in treating OUD and withdrawal with a single administration goes back to the 1960s (Alper et al., 1999). In the 1990s, the U.S. Food and Drug Administration and National Institute on Drug Abuse approved a clinical trial in humans but retracted it because of its potential cardiotoxicity (Koenig and Hilber, 2015). There are no randomized controlled trials or prospective studies on ibogaine to treat OUD, although outside the United States, several clinics provide such treatment services (Brown and Alper, 2018; Noller, Frampton, and Yazar-Klosinski, 2018).

[14] For an overview of the history of drug content testing (or "safety testing"), see MacCoun (2006).

tanyl, but how much it contains, and many tests are qualitative (i.e., they indicate whether a chemical is present) rather than quantitative (i.e., they measure how much is present).

Arguably, this creates an opportunity for a classic form of federal intervention; namely, the funding of research. Rather than being content with existing drug testing technologies, it might be possible through strategic efforts to invent or deploy new technologies that provide capabilities beyond those now available.

If methods for determining the purity of fentanyl or other synthetic opioids could be made cheaper or simpler, they might be distributed through a variety of outlets and social service outreach centers. In a 2017 study of people who use drugs in three East Coast U.S. cities, respondents thought such drug-checking services would be helpful; the majority of them reported being concerned about fentanyl and suggested that they would use such a service (Sherman et al., 2018).

Several Canadian jurisdictions offer drug-checking services to users and, perhaps, to dealers.[15] For instance, one jurisdiction in British Columbia offers advanced drug checking to clients at supervised consumption sites and other facilities (Karamouzian et al., 2018).[16] These programs not only provide users with better information regarding their drug samples, they also serve as surveillance tools, providing real-time information about what is available in local drug markets.

---

[15] The availability of drug checking to dealers is not explicitly advertised, but the services do not turn anyone away. According to interviewees familiar with these programs, one piece of evidence indicating that dealers use the service is the fact that the purity of some tested samples is too high to have been purchased at the street level.

[16] The service utilizes a combination of a Fourier-Transform Infrared (FT-IR) spectrometer and fentanyl immunoassay testing strips. Although immunoassays have a much lower sensitivity threshold than FT-IR, they are increasingly less useful as fentanyl becomes more prevalent, resulting in positive tests in most drug samples. Therefore, spectrometers are used to provide information on the concentration of fentanyl in the sample, although they are unable to detect quantities lower than 3 or 4 percent. In those instances, fentanyl strips can establish whether the concentration of fentanyl is too low to be detected by the spectrometer or whether the sample contains no fentanyl at all (Tupper et al. 2018).

Considering Supervised Consumption Sites

Supervised consumption sites allow clients to use street-purchased drugs under medical supervision. Such programs exist in Australia, Canada, and Europe; no such program has been sanctioned to operate in the United States as of this writing. Canada has made supervised consumption sites—as well as less formal versions, which are referred to as overdose prevention sites—an important part of its response to the overdose crisis (Health Canada, 2019).

Millions of drug use episodes have been supervised at such consumption sites with no reported overdose deaths; however, uncertainties remain about the magnitude of the population-level effects (Pardo, Caulkins, and Kilmer, 2018; Caulkins, Pardo, and Kilmer, 2019). The published literature on supervised consumption sites is large and generally positive, but Pardo, Caulkins, and Kilmer (2018) notes that it is limited both in nature and in the number of sites evaluated. Yet, given the longevity of some of the existing sites, it is unlikely that they would have stayed open if they resulted in significant negative outcomes for their clients or the communities where they are located. Considering the severity of the overdose crisis, some U.S. jurisdictions might decide (and have decided) that the dearth of studies that permit making causal inferences is outweighed by the apparent absence of risk, the strong face validity of these programs, and the fact that no one has died from a drug overdose at these sites.

The U.S. Department of Justice under the Trump administration argues that opening a supervised consumption site would violate federal law (Rosenstein, 2018; McSwain et al., 2019). Of course, the federal government has several options if it wished to allow such sites to operate. One option is to change the law. Another would be to treat the sites like state-legal cannabis stores (which also violate the Controlled Substances Act) and ignore them. Lastly, the federal government could publish a memo stating that supervised consumption sites will not be federal enforcement priorities under certain conditions or after taking certain steps, such as establishing local partnerships and incorporating a strong research component (Kilmer and Pardo, 2019). This last option is reminiscent of the Obama administration's response to the state-licensed cannabis industry.

Improving Supply Disruption

The transition to fentanyl and other synthetic opioids is driven by suppliers, so it makes sense to consider supply reduction as one piece of a comprehensive effort. Even if supply cannot be eliminated altogether, delaying the entrenchment of fentanyl in a market by even a few years could save hundreds, if not thousands, of lives. Yet, there is a deserved rejection of some excesses of the recent past. There is little reason to believe that tougher sentences, including drug-induced homicide laws for low-level retailers and easily replaced functionaries (e.g., couriers), will make a positive difference (see, e.g., Kleiman, 2009), There is also little reason to believe that synthetic opioid production, which occurs mostly in China, could be curtailed in the short run (Pardo, Kilmer, and Huang, 2019). However, just as there are many types of harm reduction, there are many types of supply reduction—each with its own costs and benefits. Targeting importers and wholesalers of nearly pure fentanyl from China is very different from punishing street-level retailers, who might not know the exact chemicals or purity in what they sell.

Efforts are already under way to improve technologies for detecting small shipments through the mail and parcel services (such as UPS or FedEx). USPS might improve its knowledge of the patterns of dispatch by Chinese suppliers and use its monitoring capacities more efficiently.[17] Although inventing technologies and reporting protocols that help detect fentanyl in parcels is clearly innovative and could be of great value, the longer history of drug interdiction involves an arms race of constant technological adaptation by both sides. Improved detection leads smugglers to find new importation methods to blunt the effectiveness of the new interdiction methods. Guerrero Castro (2017) refers

---

[17] Under the STOP Act of 2018, USPS is mandated to obtain advanced electronic data from packages that arrive from China. It is unclear what share of inbound packages comply with this new requirement. But, as noted in Chapter Three, the postal services of the United States and China entered into an agreement in 2011 to streamline mail delivery and reduce shipping costs for merchandise originating from China (USPS, 2011). It might make sense to revisit this agreement in light of law enforcement's assessment that a significant amount of the fentanyl and synthetic opioids being used in the United States is produced in and shipped from China.

to the "co-evolution of technology" by smugglers and interdictors. The resulting multiplicity of smuggling modes is impressive: Tunnels, drones, submarines, and concealment in frozen fruit shipments are just some of the means used to smuggle drugs. Furthermore, synthetic opioids' extreme potency and resulting small volumes help smugglers and challenge interdictors.

There could be other approaches to interdiction besides accelerating that arms race of detection and evasion technologies. Efforts could be made higher up in the supply chain to target importers and distributors who often use the internet to obtain and distribute fentanyl. For example, the DEA or another federal agency could set up phony drug-selling websites similar to what the Dutch police did with the Hansa network, to which many users migrated after the Alpha Bay crypto-market website was shut down (Europol, 2018). Some sites could make controlled deliveries to buyers who import and are likely to be dealers themselves, so they could be arrested in "reverse stings." Other DEA-operated counterfeit sites could promise—but not deliver—synthetic opioids, sending either nothing or inert powders. Even if purchasers do not face arrest, the failure of some sites to fulfill orders might lead to wariness of online procurement generally that would reduce the demand for actual fentanyl sellers.

It is hard to determine how dealers would adapt to these supply-side efforts, but the fact that some of these individuals use the internet to transact sales offers law enforcement unique insights and opportunities. Higher-level producers and distributors might move away from the surface web to the dark web if authorities continue to be successful in shutting down or seizing websites. However, it remains to be seen if dark web marketplace administrators will allow listings for fentanyl or more-potent synthetic opioids.

The government could attempt to hack or disable websites that sell drugs, or at least swamp their comment boards with phony complaints. There is no doubt that there are legal issues that we are missing, so we offer this suggestion tentatively. However, conventional interdiction has involved active disruption (e.g., crop eradication), not just reactive investigation. As the adage holds, sometimes the best defense is a good offense, so it may be worth exploring the legality and feasibility of non-traditional options of this ilk (Freeborn, 2009).

Improving Targeting of Efforts to Prevent the Spread of Synthetic Opioids

Enforcement efforts have had only limited success in shutting down established drug markets (Pollack and Reuter, 2014), but they could have somewhat more success in preventing the emergence of drug markets (Caulkins and Reuter, 2010). If that view is correct, then it might be useful to focus law enforcement on places that are about to have sudden market growth rather than places where the market is already established. Predictive analytics has provided a working substitute in many domains and is routinely tapped to improve legal supply chains (Schoenherr and Speier-Pero, 2015). It might also help to identify which counties or ZIP codes are at the highest risk of becoming fentanyl-infected and then focus resources there. This effort could tap social media data, panels of individuals who use drugs (perhaps recruited in treatment settings), wastewater testing, and a resurrected Arrestee Drug Abuse Monitoring (ADAM) program (discussed further in Appendix C).

There also could be room for tighter coupling of law enforcement deployment decisions with forensic lab reports. The goal should be to target suppliers bringing fentanyl into markets where it had previously been rare, and that requires quick feedback to police about undercover purchases or seizures with fentanyl; this should lead to an intense effort to identify and arrest the responsible distributors. Likewise, greater attention could be devoted to suppliers who mix fentanyl into other drugs besides opioids, because users of those drugs are more likely to be "opioid-naïve" and at greater risk of overdose.[18]

---

[18] At the higher levels of the distribution chain, the DEA and border control agencies might find ways (e.g., through public and private channels) of making Mexican DTOs understand that selling these products to new markets will lead to their being subject to more-intense investigation. This is similar to a suggestion that Mark Kleiman made for reducing violence in the Mexican drug trade by having the DEA target the most violent Mexican DTOs in the U.S. markets (Kleiman, 2011).

Final Thoughts

Some of the ideas mentioned in this chapter will challenge those who reject all supply disruption efforts. Other ideas may be anathema for those who believe that harm-reduction programs send the wrong message about drug consumption. That is expected, both because we intentionally included ideas that that are considered "nontraditional" throughout most of the United States and for a more fundamental reason: Our overarching message is that this crisis is different and its successful resolution will require new thinking. Prior beliefs about various drug policies might be less applicable to the current crisis. Indeed, it could be that resolution of this crisis requires approaches or technologies that do not exist today. Limiting responses to small tweaks on existing approaches in the United States will likely be insufficient and may condemn many people to early deaths.

Background Information on Synthetic Opioids

Terminology

Synthetic opioids are a broad class of drugs. Technically, synthetic opioids include any opioid (i.e., a substance that binds to opioid receptors and produces morphine-like effects) that is chemically synthesized, as opposed to being derived from the poppy plant. *Opiates* is the term used for the corresponding chemicals found in the poppy plant, notably morphine, codeine, and thebaine. Heroin is considered to be *semisynthetic* because it is synthesized from morphine, which comes from the poppy plant. Fentanyl, on the other hand, is wholly synthesized from other chemicals. The same is true of fentanyl's many analogs (sometimes referred to as *fentanyl-related substances*), such as carfentanil and sufentanil. Synthetic opioids include such prescription medications as tramadol and even medications used to treat OUD, such as methadone. Indeed, fentanyl itself is commonly used in medicine.

The number of different synthetic opioids found in drug markets is growing and ranges from substances that are less potent than morphine to those that are tens of thousands of times more potent. Some people use *fentanyl* to stand for the entire class, in part because fentanyl is by far the most common synthetic opioid in illicit drug markets in the United States. It would be similar to describing stimulant consumption in the United States using a single descriptor, without referring to the variation of such compounds as nicotine, caffeine, cocaine, methamphetamine, and cathinones.

Some data collection systems, such as MCOD records, do not distinguish among the many different synthetic opioids. MCOD does

contain a separate code for methadone, so it reports illicitly manufactured fentanyl within a broad category labeled "synthetic opioids other
than methadone" that also includes prescription tramadol, prescription
fentanyl, and such fentanyl analogs as carfentanil.

Throughout this report, we use the term *synthetic opioids* to refer
to fentanyl, its analogs, and other novel synthetic opioids that, in general, are illicitly manufactured. For the purposes of this report, we do
not use the term to refer to methadone or tramadol, which are synthesized and are often prescribed medications. Figure A.1 shows this
nomenclature.

Opioids and Morphine Equivalency

Opioids all bind to opioid receptors, including the μ-opioid receptor, in
the central nervous system. However, not all opioids work in the same
way. Some, like morphine, oxycodone, and fentanyl, are full agonists—
that is, they bind to receptors to produce a response. There also are
antagonists, which block the effects of agonists. This is what makes
the overdose reversal drug, naloxone, which is an antagonist, critical to
saving lives. It binds to opioid receptors in the brain more effectively
than do opioid agonists, such as heroin or fentanyl, thereby displacing
them and blocking their effects. Partial agonists, like buprenorphine,

Figure A.1
Nomenclature of Opioids and Examples

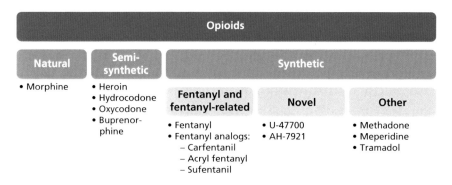

have both agonist and antagonist properties. These bind to receptors but only partially activate them and, in the presence of a competing agonist, act like an antagonist (Jackson, 2010).

The term *potency* is often used to describe the strength or concentration of a drug needed to produce a desired effect. A high-potency drug elicits an effect in lower concentrations (Atack and Lavreysen, 2010). However, drugs have various effects, so there are various measures of potency. Two measures used in pharmacology are the median effective dose (ED_{50}, or the amount needed to produce a desired response in half of the population) and the median lethal dose (LD_{50}, or the amount needed to kill half of the tested population; Neubig et al., 2003).

Because many opioids are used to treat pain, medical practitioners developed a scale to facilitate dosing of different opioids in patients (Natusch, 2012). In this context, opioids are measured relative to morphine, the first opiate extracted from the poppy plant. The MED, which is sometimes expressed in milligrams, is a useful but imprecise measure because the half-life, route of administration, and bioavailability of opioids can vary.

For example, on that scale, heroin is about two to five times as potent as morphine (Reichle et al., 1962). The median lethal dose of fentanyl in humans is not known, but generally, the reported potency ranges from 50 to 100 times that of morphine (Vardanyan and Hruby, 2014). We use the midpoint value of 75 morphine-equivalent potency for various calculations throughout this report.

Variations on the fentanyl compound have resulted in the discovery of extremely potent analogs, such as carfentanil, which is reported to be 10,000 times as potent as morphine (Vardanyan and Hruby, 2014), meaning that 0.001 mg (or 1 mcg) of carfentanil is the equivalent of 10 mg of morphine.

The Economics of Mexican Heroin and Fentanyl

This appendix provides insights about the economics of Mexican heroin and illegally produced fentanyl. Price data along the supply chain for both substances are hard to come by, especially at the retail level, where the two substances are increasingly mixed. Thus, we are forced to combine insights from various government, media, and other sources, which are sometimes contradictory or incomplete. Readers should focus more on the ranges and orders of magnitude than on specific numbers.

Heroin

Since about 2010, almost all of the heroin consumed in the United States is believed to have been produced in Mexico (DEA, 2018e). Traditionally, the heroin supply was bifurcated, with Mexican tar supplying markets west of the Mississippi River and Colombian powder supplying markets in the east; however, there has been a substantial change over the past 20 years. As documented in Sam Quinones' *Dreamland* (2015), there was a push by syndicates from Jalisco to sell more black tar east of the Mississippi River. Soon after, Mexican DTOs adopted synthesis methods used by Colombian drug producers to produce powder heroin. Colombia is now believed to play an insignificant role in the U.S. heroin market (DEA, 2018e). Although supply sources have shifted, according to the DEA, tar remains dominant in the west, while powder is more prevalent in the east, emphasizing the stickiness of market preferences.

Opium gum is the primary input to heroin manufacture, with 12 to 22 kg of opium gum being used to produce 1 kg of pure heroin (Andrés Ospina, Hernández Tinajero, and Jelsma, 2018). Over the past ten years, the price of opium gum appears to have dropped dramatically in Mexico. Mexican growers used to be able to sell 1 kg of gum to processors for more than $1,000. For example, UNODC (2018) reports that the average price per kilogram of Mexican gum was about $2,000 in 2010. Likewise, based on media reports and primary research, Andrés Ospina, Hernández Tinajero, and Jelsma (2018) reports that "[I]n the period from 2010 to 2015, years of relative economic stability, a kilo of opium gum sold for between 13,000 and 17,000 pesos in Guerrero ($1,000 to $1,250) and up to 22,000 pesos in the region of Sinaloa, Chihuahua and Durango ($1,500 to $1,600)."

However, the Network of Researchers in International Affairs reports significant previous drops from 2017 to 2018, and various media outlets report that some farmers can only get about $250 for 1 kg of opium gum (see Table B.1).[1] Of course, one needs to be very careful about taking press reports at face value, but they are suggestive of a substantial price decline, even if they cannot give very precise understanding of the magnitude of that decline.

One of the sources in Table B.1 attributes some of decline to the introduction of synthetic opioids, and this is consistent with some other accounts (e.g., Hamilton, 2019). However, there are at least two other non–mutually exclusive hypotheses that could be considered: (1) increased production is driving down prices—the United Nations reported that the area under poppy cultivation in Mexico increased 20 percent from June 2015 to July 2016 (UNODC, 2018); and (2) DTOs are starting to exert more power over the producers.

---

[1]   According to Grandmaison, Morris, and Smith (2019), "In the Sierra de Sinaloa, there has been a very similar drop off in the price offered for a kilo of opium from around 18,000 pesos ($950) in 2017 to between 8,000 pesos and 12,000 pesos ($415–$625) a kilo offered for the 2018 harvest. Oaxaca has also seen the same declining trend, from prices of around 20,000 pesos ($10,060) per kilo offered in 2017, to around 6,000 pesos ($315) a kilo offered this year." For more on this, see Bonello (2019). The value of the Mexican peso against the U.S. dollar dropped dramatically after the 2016 U.S. presidential election (Martin and Villamil, 2018) and has fluctuated for multiple reasons (Iosebashvili, 2018). This, however, does not explain the very large drop in the price of opium gum.

Table B.1
Media Reports of Opium Gum Prices in Mexico

Source	Publication Date	Price (kg)	Information Source and Location
"Opium Prices Plummet, Narcos Turn to Mining and Farmers Left in Poverty" (2018)	December 28, 2018	$180–$200	According to a church bishop in mountainous areas of Guerrero: "The price fell completely. Three years ago, [opium gum] cost 35,000 or 40,000 pesos [$1,800–$2,000] a kilo and now they're paying 3,500 or 4,000 pesos [$180–$200]. The people in the Sierra with whom I have contact don't want to plant [poppies] anymore, they say simply that 'it doesn't maintain us anymore.'"
Guthrie (2018)	August 19, 2018	$263	"But this lucrative industry is under threat. Guerrero state security spokesman Roberto Alvarez says increased use in the U.S. of synthetic opioids such as fentanyl has caused prices for Mexican opium paste on the black market to plummet to as little as $263 per kilo from more than $1,000 per kilo a year ago."
Stevenson (2018)	June 21, 2018	$250	According to Stevenson, "What has . . . farmers in the region desperate is a huge drop in the prices that local drug gangs pay for 1 kg of opium paste. At its height a few years ago, the farmers say they could get 20,000 or 25,000 pesos ($1,000–$1,250) per kilogram. This year, prices have dropped to 5,000 ($250) per kilo."

How a significant change in production costs affects prices further down the distribution chain is a long-standing debate in drug policy circles (see, e.g., Caulkins, 1990; Caulkins and Reuter, 1998). Given the dearth of data about wholesale heroin prices in Mexico in recent years, it is hard to tell a convincing story either way. The most recent report from the UNODC (2018) suggests that 1 kg of heroin at the wholesale level in Mexico circa 2015 or 2016 was $35,000. Although purity information for wholesale heroin in Mexico was not reported to UNODC, the DEA's Heroin Signature Program (HSP) reported in October 2018 that

> The average overall purity of Mexican-origin heroin analyzed through the HSP in 2016 decreased 4 percentage points, from 56 percent in 2015 to 52 percent in 2016. Within Mexican signatures, MEXSA [white powder] heroin remained highly refined with a purity level at 70 percent, followed by . . . MEX/BP [brown powder] at 44 percent; and MEX/T [black tar] at 37 percent.[2]

Unfortunately, this does not tell us much about the recent changes. In January 2019, journalist Keegan Hamilton reported that "a single kilo of regular heroin typically costs $28,000 USD to buy and ship across the border, where it sells for around $60,000 USD" (Hamilton, 2019).[3] Other sources suggest that 1 kg of heroin in the United States can cost from $20,000 to $60,000, likely depending on type, purity, distance from the Mexican border, and other factors.[4]

---

[2] DEA, 2018c, p. 4. According to the DEA (2018d),

> The HSP is one essential component of the DEA Intelligence Program to identify trends in heroin trafficking and distribution in the United States. The objective of the program is to identify and quantify the chemical components of heroin seized at U.S. ports of entry (POEs), all non-POE heroin seizures weighing more than one kilogram, randomly chosen samples, and special requests for analysis.

[3] *Regular heroin* was defined as heroin that had not yet been mixed with fentanyl. Via personal communication, Hamilton noted that the $28,000 was the import price from a Mexican supplier and that he was unsure how much of that price was for the shipping versus the product.

[4] According to Moyer, Liu, and Carr (2018), in Baltimore in 2017, the cost was implied to be $60,000 per kilogram of raw heroin. According to Lombardo and Carter (2018), in Las

The purity-adjusted price for heroin at the retail level in the United States has largely been trending down as far back as the data series goes (ONDCP, 2016; Midgette et al., 2019). Although there have been temporary increases, the 2016 price per pure gram of heroin at the retail level was at the lowest level recorded: approximately $750 (in 2018 dollars), or roughly one-third of what it was 20 years earlier, after adjusting for inflation (ONDCP, 2016; Midgette et al., 2019).[5]

However, it is not entirely clear what has happened to heroin prices since 2012. None of the standard methods of tracking drug prices is designed to handle a situation in which a primary drug (in this case, heroin) routinely appears in a mixture with another drug that has similar effects, let alone when that is happening in one part of the country but not in another and the goal is to report national prices. Furthermore, there appears to be a discrepancy in two estimates of heroin price trends in the years after fentanyl's arrival. In 2018, the DEA published a chart indicating that heroin prices largely declined from 2012 to 2014 and then significantly increased from 2014 to 2016 (DEA, 2018a; see Figure B.1). It is unclear how these figures were calculated or whether they are adjusted for inflation (although inflation was quite low in those years). In contrast, estimates produced for ONDCP by RAND (Midgette et al., 2019) suggest that the price per pure gram of heroin at the retail level decreased throughout this period (2012 = $924; 2013 = $795; 2014 = $800; 2015 = $758; 2016 = $750; all values in 2018 dollars). The methodology for the latter approach is described by Arkes et al. (2004). Of course, in addition to the challenges peculiar to tracing heroin prices after fentanyl's arrival, there are perennial challenges in estimating drug market prices; however, the differences in trends are not insubstantial and deserve additional analysis.

Vegas in 2017, black tar heroin was reported to cost $26,000–$31,000 per kilogram, while brown heroin was reported to cost $21,000–$33,000 per kilogram.

[5] ONDCP (2016) reports the average retail price per gram in 1996 was $725 (2012 dollars) and purity was 37 percent. Converting to 2018 dollars ($854) and dividing by 0.37 = $2,308.

Figure B.1
**Quarterly Purity-Adjusted Heroin Prices from the DEA, January 2012–
December 2016**

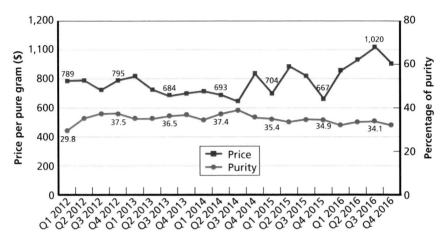

SOURCE: Adapted from DEA, 2018a.

Fentanyl

Although fentanyl is a legitimate medical product in the United States, diversion or theft from legal suppliers is not believed to account for much of the overdose problem (Gladden, Martinez, and Seth, 2016). The fentanyl and other synthetic opioids involved in overdoses generally make their way to the United States directly from China or over the border from Canada or Mexico. In the high-level market before entering the United States, recent RAND research identified multiple Chinese firms that are willing to ship 1 kg of nearly pure fentanyl to the United States for $2,000 to $5,000 (Pardo, Davis, and Moore, forthcoming).[6]

The fentanyl coming from Mexico is either imported from China or is produced in Mexico with precursors that were imported from China. Hamilton (2019) notes that:

---

[6] It is unclear, however, whether the purchased product will be shipped directly from China or one of its U.S. storage facilities.

According to sources involved in the drug trade in Culiacán, Sinaloa, who spoke to VICE News on the condition of anonymity, cartel cooks charge as little as $2,000 per kilo (for fentanyl). Pure kilos of fentanyl are said to sell to mid-level dealers in Culiacán for around $45,000, then [are] mixed with heroin and stretched into eight or nine kilos of blended product, which retail for $35,000 per kilo in Los Angeles or over $50,000 USD on the East Coast. And those are just wholesale prices—the profits increase exponentially when the kilos are further diluted and sold in smaller doses on the street.

Interestingly, according to federal law enforcement, very little of the heroin seized at the southwest border is mixed with fentanyl (CBP, 2019b; DEA, 2018e). Although it might be the case that those who are smuggling mixed products take greater precautions, it could also be the case that mixing in Mexico is uncommon.[7]

It is very difficult to track what is happening with fentanyl prices at the retail level because it is often mixed with heroin, and many users (and sellers) have no idea how much fentanyl or other synthetic opioids are in a given bag.

Trying to Compare Heroin and Fentanyl Prices

Synthetic opioids coming from China are cheaper than Mexican heroin on a purity-adjusted basis (see, e.g., DEA, 2017b; Mars, Rosenblum, and Ciccarone, 2018; Rothberg and Stith, 2018), but fair comparisons should also adjust for potency.

A construct called the morphine-equivalent dose (MED; See Appendix A) allows physicians and patients to use a common measure to compare across opioids. With MED, the strength of other drugs is relative to morphine. For example, if a substance is believed to be three times as strong as morphine per milligram, its MED would be three. Alternatively, if morphine was believed to be three times stron-

---

[7]   Lombardo and Carter (2018) notes that investigations reflect a fentanyl price of $30,000–$40,000 per kg, but information about potency was not provided.

ger than a given substance, the latter's MED would be 0.33. The MED for heroin is 2–5 and for fentanyl, the MED can range from 50 to 100 (Vardanyan and Hruby, 2014).

In terms of the MED-adjusted import price immediately before entering the United States, a 95-percent pure kg of fentanyl at $5,000 would conservatively equate to a cost of approximately $100 per MED kg.[8] For comparison, 1 kg of 50-percent pure heroin that costs $25,000 before being shipped across the U.S.-Mexico border could equate to approximately $10,000 per MED kg—which is 100 times more expensive than fentanyl in terms of MED at the import level.[9] This ratio is conservative; the discrepancy would be even larger if one believed that the heroin purity was lower or the wholesale price was higher in Mexico, if the price for fentanyl was less than $5,000, or if the MED for heroin was lower than five (or that of fentanyl was higher than 50).

---

[8] For example, $5,000 / (1 kg fentanyl × 95-percent purity × 50 to convert to MED) = $105.26. Fifty is the lower bound for the fentanyl MED.

[9] For example, $25,000 / (1 kg heroin × 50-percent purity × 5 to convert to MED) = $10,000. Five is the upper bound for the heroin MED. Using the lower bound for fentanyl and the upper bound for heroin produces a conservative estimate of the price differential.

Opportunities for Better Surveillance and Monitoring

Governments have a unique responsibility for funding data collection and monitoring of drug use, drug problems, and drug markets. On that score, the U.S. government has failed and failed badly. Whereas the United States once boasted the world's best data infrastructure for supporting evidence-informed decisionmaking, it now lags behind. For example, many other countries now routinely test wastewater to track drug consumption trends (EMCDDA, 2019d). The United States does not do that systematically.

The HIV/AIDS crisis prompted large-scale investments in new data and monitoring systems, such as the National HIV Behavioral Surveillance system. The overdose epidemic, which now kills more than HIV/AIDS did at its peak, has not elicited any comparable investment in data infrastructure.

The failure is particularly severe on the supply side. Although substantial resources go into research and monitoring with respect to health issues, much less effort is devoted to understanding the behavior of suppliers or measuring such fundamental parameters as prices and quantities. Existing systems do not even permit accurate estimation of purity-adjusted prices of fentanyl or fentanyl-adulterated heroin, at either the retail or wholesale levels.

In this appendix, we offer a few suggestions for partially remedying this unfortunate situation.

Enhancing Drug Toxicology Assessments

The federal government, through CDC, is working to improve the capacity of the states to report overdose deaths in an accurate and timely manner. The State Unintentional Drug Overdose Reporting System works to capture detailed information on toxicology, death scene investigations, route of administration, and other risk factors associated with drug overdose. As we described briefly in Chapter Two, state and local medical examiners and coroners might not always have the appropriate protocols or referent material to determine the cause of death in a drug overdose, at least in a timely and accurate way.

Toxicology screens of tissue and fluid samples, as well as analytical detection methods used to analyze seizures, can only test vis-à-vis a known universe of metabolites or chemicals. New chemical profiles are added to referent libraries once they are detected. It is plausible that early measurements of novel synthetics are biased downward, given that analytical techniques to detect them must be developed and disseminated. For example, one study sponsored by ONDCP found that initial screens of urine collected from a sample ($n = 175$) of emergency department patients in Maryland tested negative for synthetic cannabinoids. The specimens were retested later with an expanded panel and 25 percent were positive for the presence of these more-novel synthetic cannabinoids (Wish et al., 2018). Therefore, routinized retesting of postmortem biological samples could help shed light on the scope and magnitude of this problem.

In addition, current mortality data reported by CDC uses the ICD-10 coding system, which lumps all synthetic opioid overdose deaths (except methadone) into a single code. Examination of overdose deaths using a single poisoning code is rather limiting. Some states report overdoses by type of synthetic opioid, which would permit more-nuanced analysis. Including the chemical involved in synthetic opioid overdoses would enhance understanding of how these markets are evolving.

Improving the Understanding of Drug Market Actors in the Era of Fentanyl and Other Synthetic Opioids

The potency of fentanyl and other synthetic opioids is changing how sellers and buyers go about conducting business or using drugs that might contain these substances. Improving the way drug market actors respond to fentanyl's arrival will enhance policy responses.

Currently, the DEA's FSPP suggests that law enforcement is only considering two synthesis methods when analyzing fentanyl seizures. As discussed in Chapter Three, there have been several additional synthesis routes detailed in the literature. Most still start with NPP, but several point to the use of other starting or intermediate chemicals. An improved understanding of which synthesis route is utilized could offer additional insights into the supply of fentanyl and other synthetic opioids. Law enforcement indicates that there is wide disparity in the purity of fentanyl arriving at mail facilities versus the fentanyl smuggled over the border, indicating possible variations in synthesis techniques. Being able to determine synthesis profiles could help law enforcement investigate supply sources, as well as ascertain the impact of precursor controls. For example, recently published synthesis methods that start with N-benzyl-4-piperidone might offer manufacturers an avenue to circumvent restrictions on NPP (Walz and Hsu, 2017).

The DEA's long-standing assertion that Colombian heroin continued to make its way to retail markets in the eastern half of the United States as late as 2012, when in fact Mexican drug traffickers had figured out the Colombian powder recipe, is just one example of the limits of signature profiling.[1] Federal law enforcement should consider these limitations, as well as the possibility that manufacturers are using a wider variety of synthesis methods beyond the traditional Janssen and Siegfried routes.

Understanding dealer decisionmaking is also critical for understanding the market and formulating innovative and effective policy

---

[1] What is particularly striking about that continued identification of Colombia as a source was that other parts of the DEA produced estimates that Colombian heroin production had sunk to negligible levels by about 2005 (U.S. State Department, 2012).

interventions. Thus, an important task is to gain insights into how dealers who acquire synthetic opioids from the internet determine which chemical they choose to purchase and how much they put into the heroin they sell or counterfeit tablets they press; cocaine needs to be considered separately. A simple economic model of the heroin market suggests that profit-maximizing dealers would substitute cheap fentanyl for expensive heroin roughly up to the point at which the user notices a decline in the quality of the experience, assuming that quality differences can be perceived. One reason that a simple model of dealer behavior might have failed so far is that fentanyl is probably not readily available to all heroin retailers. Many heroin retailers are not web savvy and might not be able to obtain cryptocurrency or other means for purchasing remotely. Other dealers might be intimidated by the difficulty of dosing accurately with fentanyl. Some heroin dealers might not want to put their regular customers at high risk of a fatal overdose out of a mix of humanitarian and commercial concerns.

There also could be differential legal risks. The calculus underlying dealer decisions about how much to substitute fentanyl (or some other potent synthetic opioid) for heroin remains unknown; however, this calculus will determine the future pattern of such overdoses. Studies of street dealers have a long history of producing insights about the operation of markets (Johnson et al., 2018; Reuter et al., 1990). In that vein, interviews with dealers at various levels of supply (e.g., bulk importers, darknet distributors, and street dealers) would provide much-needed insight into the decisionmaking and operational processes of suppliers in markets affected by fentanyl or other synthetic opioids.[2]

For decades, the DEA has collected data on the price and purity of drugs purchased in undercover buys and the purity of seizures analyzed in federal laboratories in an administrative dataset known as the System To Retrieve Information about Drug Evidence (STRIDE, which has now been reinvented as STARLiMS). These price and purity

---

[2]   Examples of literature offering insights based on interviews with dealers include Caulkins, Burnett, and Leslie (2009); Caulkins et al. (2016); Caulkins, Gurga, and Little (2009); Desroches (2007); Dorn et al. (2005); and Reuter and Haaga (1989).

data have been a mainstay for empirical research in drug markets, but they have been made decreasingly available to researchers.

As noted in Chapter Two, NFLIS collects results of forensic tests of seized drugs for many state and local law enforcement agencies; however, only aggregate-level reports—such as the share of all cocaine samples that also contained a synthetic opioid—are made public. Now that there is a broad suite of opioids, not just heroin, and those opioids are showing up in packages of cocaine, it is important to start reporting counts of the various mixtures and combinations, not just total counts by chemical. Much could be learned by making the incident-level data available for research purposes, with appropriate privacy protections, such as the removal of exact dates and locations.

Additionally, efforts should be made to learn from user experiences. This is particularly true for those who are at risk of overdose and are most likely to come into regular contact with synthetic opioids (Mars, Ondocsin, and Ciccarone, 2018b). Many of these individuals engage with dealers, providing additional insights into retail supply trends. These studies might be enhanced with the provision of fentanyl testing strips (or other to-be-developed technologies) aimed at enhancing users' knowledge of the drugs they consume (Sherman et al., 2018). Understanding how individuals who use drugs adapt to elevated overdose risk might allow for more-targeted policy innovation as well as identify and overcome barriers to services and tools that might save lives (Park et al., 2019; Rouhani et al., 2019). Early research by Rouhani and colleagues (2019) suggests that some individuals who use drugs might take greater precautions if they were informed about the risks of fentanyl in the drugs they purchased on the street.

The possible mixing of fentanyl and other synthetic opioids into the supply of cocaine raises different problems and potential research opportunities. In 2017, synthetic opioids were found in about as many fatal overdoses when combined with cocaine as when they were combined with heroin. Deliberate mixing is one possible explanation. As discussed in Daly (2019), these mixtures might also be the consequence of cocaine users who separately buy fentanyl-contaminated heroin or of cocaine dealers carelessly handling fentanyl-contaminated heroin before they package cocaine. It is plausible that all three play a role;

analysis of seizures and undercover purchases is one path forward to understanding this.

Getting Serious About Wastewater Testing to Track Synthetic Opioids

Novel approaches to measuring drug consumption might be needed, especially in light of the fact that many fentanyl analogs and other synthetic opioids quickly enter and exit markets. Users themselves might not know that they consumed a synthetic opioid, let alone be able to point to which compound was supplied. Wastewater testing is another approach for monitoring the spread of new psychoactive substances and for measuring consumption (Castiglioni, 2016).

This technique, which is utilized in Europe—and, to a much lesser extent, in the United States—can supplement traditional epidemiological drug indicators (such as prevalence rates or overdoses). For example, wastewater analysis in Washington state found sharp increases in cannabis consumption after legalization (Burgard et al., 2019) and, in Oregon, it shows that higher concentrations of drug metabolites were found in municipalities that reported higher rates of drug use (Banta-Green et al., 2009). Cities in Europe have been developing and deploying this technique for decades, with demonstrated success in delivering near-real-time information about shifting use patterns in drug markets (Castiglioni, 2016). For example, results from one wastewater examination of eight cities in Europe found high correlations between results from tested water samples and various indicators of local drug markets, including the sales of pharmaceuticals and illicit drug seizure records (Baz-Lomba et al., 2016). A 2018 report from Australia found that fentanyl consumption, although low to begin with, might have doubled outside of capital city jurisdictions from April 2017 to April 2018 (Australian Criminal Intelligence Commission, 2018). However, such an approach might work only in areas with high connectivity to municipal water systems.

Resurrecting Some Version of the Arrestee Drug Abuse Monitoring Program

The ADAM program collected rich drug market data (including urinalysis results) from thousands of individuals arrested and jailed for any offense. In the early 2000s, ADAM covered more than 40 counties (almost exclusively urban), and there were plans to expand the program to 75 counties. The program was cut in 2003 and a much smaller version was brought back in 2007, only to be fully eliminated after 2013. Although the ADAM program did not test for fentanyl and novel synthetic opioids, it would not have been hard to incorporate this as deaths began to take off after 2013. As with wastewater testing, ADAM's biological testing could serve as an early warning and monitoring system. One also could imagine modules that ask people who use and/or sell heroin about their experiences and decisions around fentanyl and other synthetic opioids.

Multiple researchers (Kilmer and Caulkins, 2014; Kleiman, 2004; Midgette et al., 2019), as well as the Presidential Commission on Combating Drug Addiction and the Opioid Crisis (Christie et al., 2017), have called for the resurrection of some version of the ADAM program. At its peak, ADAM cost about one-fifth of what is spent each year on the NSDUH—which is not very useful for understanding heroin and illicit opioid markets (Caulkins et al., 2015). Given the billions of dollars the administration is devoting to reducing opioid overdoses, using a very small percentage of this to reconstitute ADAM seems like a very wise investment.

Improving Estimates of Opioid-Misusing Populations and Other Relevant Individual-Level Risk Factors

Greater precision of population estimates and improved knowledge of individual-level outcomes are crucial to enhancing policy responses. For example, improving the precision of estimates of people who use heroin and other opioids is paramount for focusing resources on averting potential harms generated by fentanyl and other potent synthetic opioids. It is well known that population estimates generated by NSDUH suffer from imprecision and are likely to undercount heavy heroin users who fall outside the sampling frame (Caulkins et al., 2015). Although ONDCP has funded outside research organizations to generate a more accurate estimate of this population for three decades, the elimination of ADAM requires that this methodology be radically revised.

Although reviving some version of ADAM and implementing wastewater testing can improve national, state, and substate estimates, longitudinal public health studies of at-risk drug-using populations are increasingly needed to assess important parameters of fatal and non-fatal overdose risk, as well as changing user behavior in light of transitioning markets. For example, the prospective cohort study of AIDS Linked to the IntraVenous Experience at Johns Hopkins University and the Vancouver Injection Drug Users Study provide useful models with which to gauge overdose risk and fentanyl exposure. Both of these cohort studies have been used to understand point-in-time overdose risk and response in vulnerable populations (Hayashi et al., 2018; Pollini et al., 2006). Research efforts should be made to examine and learn from the experiences of people who use drugs and face such harms.

Supplemental Information on Data and Methods

This appendix is largely reproduced from Pardo et al. (2019).

Mortality Data

Mortality data are available from CDC's National Vital Statistics System. Data for 2005 through 2017 were provided to RAND researchers under a data use agreement with CDC and contain individual death certificate records on the decedent's county of residence and information on relevant ICD-10 codes for drug poisonings. In order to examine state and county trends, we extracted drug overdose deaths with the underlying cause of death codes: unintentional (X40–X44), suicide (X60–X64), homicide (X85), and undetermined (Y10–Y14) and multiple cause of death T-codes by drug or drug class: (heroin: T40.1; natural and semisynthetic opioids [generally considered to be prescription opioids]: T40.2; methadone: T40.3; synthetic opioids other than methadone: T40.4; cocaine: T40.5; and unknown/unspecified drug: T50.9). In the state-level analyses, we have suppressed jurisdiction-years with fewer than ten deaths from data visualizations.

Summary counts of overdoses across drug categories are not mutually exclusive. For example, an individual who consumed heroin tainted with fentanyl would show up in counts involving heroin as well as those involving synthetic opioids. Therefore, analyses that only examine total counts by drug often ignore the share of overdoses that co-involve other substances. Because we have access to individual death records, we can calculate the share of overdose deaths by jurisdiction-

year that mention synthetic opioids alone and in combination with various other drug categories.

CDC's National Center for Health Statistics, in collaboration with the U.S. Census Bureau, reports annual population estimates by counties via the Bridged-Race Resident Population Estimates online tool (CDC, 2019). From this, we obtained county and state population estimates in order to calculate unadjusted or crude overdose death rates. Spencer et al. (2019) notes that the crude and age-adjusted rates of overdose deaths involving fentanyl from 2011 to 2016 were similar.

Some overdose death cases do not list a specific drug. Nationally, the percentage of overdose deaths not listing a specific drug declined from 22 percent to 12 percent from 2013 to 2017. However, several states that have been severely affected by fatal drug overdoses moved in the opposite direction and have reported sharp rises in the number of deaths categorized as unspecified or unknown. This suggests that there might be undercounting of overdoses caused by synthetic opioids or other drugs (Ruhm, 2018), perhaps because medical examiners were simply overwhelmed by the increased workload or lacked resources, including up-to-date referent material, to accurately determine the underlying cause of death.[1]

Given the potential measurement error in drug death reporting, we have restricted state-level analysis to states that, according to Scholl et al. (2018), have very good to excellent overdose reporting in 2017 (see Table D.1). These states include Ohio, West Virginia, and states in New England.

Seizure Data

We draw from publicly available law enforcement reports and congressional testimonies (namely, those from the DEA and CBP). Such

---

[1] Pennsylvania could be a constructive example. Its uncategorized overdose deaths were stable between 2005 and 2013 but doubled after 2014, when fentanyl started to appear in neighboring states. The number of uncategorized overdoses in Pennsylvania now outnumbers overdose fatalities that involve heroin or synthetic opioids by factors of three and 1.25, respectively.

Table D.1
Overdose Reporting Quality by State, 2017

Very Good to Excellent		Good	Fair	
Alaska	North Carolina	Arizona[a]	Alabama	Mississippi
Connecticut	Ohio[b]	California[a]	Arkansas	Montana
District of Columbia[a]	Oklahoma	Colorado	Delaware	North Dakota
Georgia[b]	Oregon	Kentucky[a]	Florida	Nebraska
Hawaii[a]	Rhode Island	Michigan[a]	Idaho	New Jersey
Illinois[b]	South Carolina	Minnesota	Indiana	Pennsylvania
Iowa	Tennessee[b]	Missouri	Kansas	South Dakota
Maine	Utah	Texas[a]	Louisiana	Wyoming
Maryland	Vermont			
Massachusetts	Virginia			
Nevada	Washington			
New Hampshire	West Virginia			
New Mexico	Wisconsin			
New York				

SOURCE: Scholl et al., 2018.
[a] Denotes "fair" reporting in 2014 for states that CDC did not consider to be fair in 2017.
[b] Denotes "good" reporting in 2014 for states that CDC did not consider to be good in 2017.

reports and testimonies provide a general overview of the volume of seizures over time, their likely sources of origin, and illicit actors involved.

We used laboratory seizure data from NFLIS to provide insights into where and when specific synthetic opioids enter and exit drug markets. NFLIS systematically collects drug chemistry analysis results and other related information from cases analyzed by state, local, and federal forensic laboratories. Partner laboratories examine drug seizures secured by law enforcement across the country. According to the DEA, almost all state and local crime laboratories now participate in NFLIS.

Nevertheless, limitations remain in using these data. Public law enforcement and forensics data lack granular details. For example, NFLIS seizure case counts are aggregated to the state level and do not report purity or the proportion of fentanyl-containing seizures that are mixed with other drugs, such as heroin.

More importantly, seizures are not random samples of the supply of drugs. They are convenience samples that might depend on factors related to law enforcement priority, capacity, and targeting. Given rising overdose deaths from synthetic overdoses, it is likely that law enforcement at every level (federal, state, and local) have prioritized these drug threats in recent years. Therefore, seizure incidents could be confounded by political pressures or policy directives. With traditional drugs, such as cocaine or heroin, it has been challenging to determine the underlying factors that contribute to an increase (or decrease) in seizures from one year to the next (Reuter, 1995). Law enforcement capacity and the intensity of efforts to detect and seize illicit drug shipments, as well as the ability and determination of smugglers to evade detection, could vary over time in ways that confound analysis of seizure trends.

Details on Key Informant Interviews

Key informant interviews were one of the two principal inputs inform-ing the international experience with fentanyl discussion in Chap-ter Four. We interviewed individuals who were knowledgeable about synthetic opioids in selected international jurisdictions and/or aspects of fentanyl markets in general. Informants included the following stakeholder groups: (1) public officials working in the areas of drug policy or public health surveillance; for example, individuals working for national ministries with illicit drugs in their portfolios (e.g., health, social affairs, interior) and for national monitoring bodies; (2) public health professionals (e.g., practitioners working for a medical facility or for an organization providing services to PWUD); (3) law enforcement professionals (e.g., practitioners working for local, regional, or national police agencies) and customs officials; and (4) researchers working on various aspects of drug policy. In total, we conducted 22 interviews involving 25 key informants. Table E.1 provides a breakdown of key informants by stakeholder group. Table E.2 offers a breakdown of interviewees by country.

In a few instances, interviewees offered to consult with their colleagues and professional networks on any questions raised during the interviews. It is impossible to account for these additional con-sulted individuals in this appendix, although we are grateful for their contributions.

Table E.1
Key Informants, by Stakeholder Group

Stakeholder Group	Number of Interviewees
Drug policy or surveillance	9
Law enforcement	9
Public health professional	4
Researcher	3
Total	25

NOTE: Each interviewee was assigned to only one stakeholder group, corresponding to the person's primary occupation. However, multiple interviewees could plausibly be categorized in multiple ways. For instance, numerous public health professionals also hold academic positions and engage in research.

Table E.2
Key Informants, by Country

Country	Number of Interviewees
Canada	8
Estonia	6
Finland	3
Latvia	2
Sweden	3
Other	3
Total	25

NOTE: In addition to commenting on the drug market in their respective countries, interviewees were invited to share insights on the situation in other countries. "Other" refers to interviewees who were not from any of the focus countries.

Recruitment

Interviewees were identified either via the research team's professional networks or via literature review. The desk review focused on, but was not limited to, individuals who have published on the topic of national drug markets or have been affiliated with relevant institutions in focus countries (e.g., governmental organizations with competencies in the area of drug policy, law enforcement bodies, or public health surveillance organizations). We also employed a snowballing approach to recruitment; we asked each interviewee for recommendations for additional individuals to consult. In all cases, potential interviewees were approached via email using standardized invitation language, followed by additional email and phone contact as necessary.

Execution

Interviews were conducted by phone. At the beginning of each session, interviewees were provided with information about the purpose of the interview and how information collected during the conversation would be used. We obtained verbal consent for audio-recording. These recordings were used to update and finalize contemporaneous notes taken by researchers.

Interviews were semistructured and followed a unified general topic guide consisting of broad questions to be covered by each interview (see "the Interview Topic Guide" section). At the same time, the topic guide allowed for a discussion of unanticipated topics, was complemented by questions tailored to the specific country context, and allowed interviewees to address questions raised in the data collection process.

Analysis

Information collected via key informant interviews was incorporated in individual country overviews as appropriate. This process focused on complementing information collected from official documentation with facts and insights provided by the interviewees. For our comparative analysis, which brings together lessons from all focus countries, we employed standard principles of qualitative data analysis. We explored interview notes for commonalities and divergences across interviews and identified insights for inclusion in the comparative analysis. These insights were organized into individual themes, to which relevant parts of interview notes were assigned. These themes, in turn, formed the basis for the structure of the remainder of Chapter Four.

Interview Topic Guide

[tailored according to the context of each interviewee's country]

1. Could you briefly describe your role and responsibilities?
   a. [*prompts: how long have you been in your post?*]
2. How would you describe the situation regarding fentanyl in [JURISDICTION]?
   a. [*prompts: How big a role does fentanyl play? What are the data on fentanyl supply and demand?*]
3. What is the source of fentanyl? How is it distributed?
   a. [*prompts: Has this changed over time? Does this differ between fentanyl and its analogs? Is there any domestic illicit production of fentanyl?*]
4. How is fentanyl sold in [JURISDICTION]?
   a. [*prompts: What form is fentanyl typically in (e.g., powder, nasal spray, counterfeit pills)? How is it administered?*]
5. What is the purity and price of fentanyl and/or analogs?
   a. [*prompts: How expensive is fentanyl compared with other opioids?*]
6. Are other opioids available in [JURISDICTION]?
   a. [*prompts: How do these markets coexist with the fentanyl market? Is fentanyl mixed with heroin? Why or why not?*]
7. Can fentanyl be prescribed in [JURISDICTION]?
   a. [*prompts: Has there been documented diversion of medically dispensed fentanyl?*]
8. What are the current trends in the fentanyl market?
   a. [*prompts: Is the fentanyl market stable? What do you expect the future developments to be? Why?*]
9. Has fentanyl been reported to be mixed with heroin? With other drugs?
   a. [*prompts: Is there any explanation for why or why not?*]
10. Could you describe how fentanyl arrived in [JURISDICTION]?
    a. [*prompts: When did fentanyl enter the country? How quickly, if at all, did it displace heroin?*]

11. Were there any factors that can help explain the arrival of fentanyl?
    a. [*prompts: Demand-side factors? Supply-side factors?*]
12. Did fentanyl start serving an existing user population?
    a. [*prompts: Is there any evidence that it created its own demand?*]
13. What is known about users' preferences and perspectives on fentanyl?
    a. [*prompts: Are they aware of what is happening in the market? Have they adapted to the arrival of fentanyl? How?*]
14. How, if at all, does the situation in [JURISDICTION] compare with that in other countries?
    a. [*prompts: Do you have any thoughts on why the situation differs from other countries in the region? What are the specificities of the market in (JURISDICTION)?*]
15. Is there something else you would like to comment on?
16. Is there someone else you think we should speak with for this study?
17. Is there any documentation or data you think would be helpful for the research team to review?

Thank you very much for your time.

References

Ahmad, F. B., L. A. Escobedo, L. M. Rossen, M. R. Spencer, M. Warner, and P. Sutton, *Provisional Drug Overdose Death Counts*, Hyattsville, Md.: National Center for Health Statistics, 2019. As of July 11, 2019:
https://www.cdc.gov/nchs/nvss/vsrr/drug-overdose-data.htm

Akerlof, George A., "The Market for 'Lemons': Quality Uncertainty and the Market Mechanism," *Quarterly Journal of Economics*, Vol. 84, No. 3, August 1970, pp. 488–500. As of July 11, 2019:
https://www2.bc.edu/thomas-chemmanur/phdfincorp/MF891%20papers/Ackerlof%201970.pdf

Aldridge, Judith, and David Décary-Hétu, "Not an 'Ebay for Drugs': the Cryptomarket 'Silk Road' as a Paradigm Shifting Criminal Innovation," *SSRN*, May 13, 2014.

Aldridge, Judith, and David Décary-Hétu, "Hidden Wholesale: The Drug Diffusing Capacity of Online Drug Cryptomarkets," *International Journal of Drug Policy*, Vol. 35, September 2016, pp. 7–15.

Alho, Hannu, David Sinclair, Erkki Vuori, and Antti Holopainen, "Abuse Liability of Buprenorphine–Naloxone Tablets in Untreated IV Drug Users," *Drug and Alcohol Dependence*, Vol. 88, No. 1, 2007, pp. 75–78.

Allday, Erin, "Fentanyl Rising as Killer in San Francisco—57 Dead in a Year," *San Francisco Chronicle*, June 23, 2019. As of July 11, 2019:
https://www.sfchronicle.com/health/article/Fentanyl-rising-as-killer-in-San-Francisco-57-14030821.php?psid=ci5BX

Alper, Kenneth R., Howard S. Lotsof, Geerte M. N. Frenken, Daniel J. Luciano, and Jan Bastiaans, "Treatment of Acute Opioid Withdrawal with Ibogaine," *American Journal on Addictions*, Vol. 8, No. 3, 1999, pp. 234–242.

Alpert, Abby, David Powell, and Rosalie Liccardo Pacula, *Supply-Side Drug Policy in the Presence of Substitutes: Evidence from the Introduction of Abuse-Deterrent Opioids*, Cambridge, Mass.: National Bureau of Economic Research, NBER Working Paper No. 23031, January 2017. As of July 11, 2019: https://www.nber.org/papers/w23031

Amlani, Ashraf, Geoff McKee, Noren Khamis, Geetha Raghukumar, Erica Tsang, and Jane A. Buxton, "Why the FUSS (Fentanyl Urine Screen Study)? A Cross-Sectional Survey to Characterize an Emerging Threat to People Who Use Drugs in British Columbia, Canada," *Harm Reduction Journal*, Vol. 12, No. 54, 2015.

Andrés Ospina, Guillermo, Jorge Hernández Tinajero, and Martin Jelsma, *Poppies, Opium and Heroin: Production in Colombia and Mexico*, Amsterdam, The Netherlands: Transnational Institute, February 2018. As of July 23, 2019: https://www.tni.org/files/publication-downloads/poppiesopiumheroin_13042018_web.pdf

Arkes, Jeremy, Rosalie Liccardo Pacula, Susan Paddock, Jonathan P. Caulkins, and Peter Reuter, *Technical Report for the Price and Purity of Illicit Drugs: 1981 Through the Second Quarter of 2003*, Washington, D.C.: Office of National Drug Control Policy, November 2004. As of July 23, 2019: https://obamawhitehouse.archives.gov/sites/default/files/ondcp/policy-and-research/bullet_4.pdf

Armenian, Patil, Kathy T. Vo, Jill Barr-Walker, and Kara L. Lynch, "Fentanyl, Fentanyl Analogs and Novel Synthetic Opioids: A Comprehensive Review," *Neuropharmacology*, Vol. 134, 2018, pp. 121–132.

Armenian Patil, Jeffrey D. Whitman, Adina Badea, Whitney Johnson, Chelsea Drake, Simranjit Singh Dhillon, Michelle Rivera, Nicklaus Brandehoff, and Kara L. Lynch, "*Notes from the Field*: Unintentional Fentanyl Overdoses Among Persons Who Thought They Were Snorting Cocaine—Fresno, California, January 7, 2019," *Morbidity and Mortality Weekly Report*, Vol. 68, No. 31, 2019, pp. 687–688. As of August 20, 2019: https://www.cdc.gov/mmwr/volumes/68/wr/mm6831a2.htm

"Aseguran en Culiacán, Sinaloa presunto laboratorio de fentanilo," Debate.com, April 11, 2019. As of July 11, 2019: https://www.debate.com.mx/policiacas/Aseguran-en-Culiacan-Sinaloa-presunto-laboratorio-de-fentanilo-20190411-0095.html

Atack, John, and Hilde Lavreysen, "Agonist," in P. Stolerman, ed., *Encyclopedia of Psychopharmacology*, Heidelberg, Germany: Springer-Verlag Berlin Heidelberg, 2010, p. 45.

Australian Criminal Intelligence Commission, *National Wastewater Drug Monitoring Program: Report 6*, Canberra, Australia, December 2018. As of July 11, 2019: https://www.acic.gov.au/sites/default/files/2019/02/ww6_300119.pdf?v=1561684377

Australian Injecting and Illicit Drug Users League, *Injecting Fentanyl: Minimising the Risks*, Canberra, Australia, 2013. As of July 11, 2019:
http://www.aivl.org.au/wp-content/uploads/2018/05/
Injecting-Fentanyl-Minimising-The-Risks.pdf

Australian Institute of Health and Welfare, *Opioid Harm in Australia and Comparisons Between Australia and Canada*, Canberra, Australia, 2018. As of July 11, 2019:
https://www.aihw.gov.au/getmedia/
605a6cf8-6e53-488e-ac6e-925e9086df33/aihw-hse-210.pdf.aspx?inline=true

Babor, Thomas F., Jonathan P. Caulkins, Griffith Edwards, Benedikt Fischer, David R. Foxcroft, Keith Humphreys, Isidore S. Obot, Jürgen Rehm, Peter Reuter, Robin Room, Ingeborg Rossow, and John Strang, *Drug Policy and the Public Good*, 2nd ed., New York: Oxford University Press, 2018.

Baker, Rafferty, "New Program Will Distribute Free Opioids to Entrenched Users," MSN news, January 4, 2019. As of July 23, 2019:
https://www.msn.com/en-ca/news/canada/
new-program-will-distribute-free-opioids-to-entrenched-users/ar-BBRNkl8

Baldwin, Nicholas, Roger Gray, Anirudh Goel, Evan Wood, Jane A. Buxton, and Launette Marie Rieb, "Fentanyl and Heroin Contained in Seized Illicit Drugs and Overdose-Related Deaths in British Columbia, Canada: An Observational Analysis," *Drug and Alcohol Dependence*, Vol. 185, 2018, pp. 322–327.

Banta-Green, Caleb J., Jennifer A. Field, Aurea C. Chiaia, Daniel L. Sudakin, Laura Power, and Luc de Montigny, "The Spatial Epidemiology of Cocaine, Methamphetamine and MDMA Use: A Demonstration Using a Population Measure of Community Drug Load Derived from Municipal Wastewater," *Addiction*, Vol. 104, No. 11, 2009, pp. 1874–1880.

Barratt, Monica J., "Silk Road: Ebay for Drugs: The Journal Publishes Both Invited and Unsolicited Letters," *Addiction*, Vol. 107, No. 3, 2012, pp. 683–683.

Baz-Lomba, Jose Antonio, Stefania Salvatore, Emma Gracia-Lor, Richard Bade, Sara Castiglioni, Erika Castrignanò, Ana Causanilles, Felix Hernandez, Barbara Kasprzyk-Hordern, Juliet Kinyua, Ann-Kathrin McCall, Alexander van Nuijs, Christoph Ort, Benedek G. Plósz, Pedram Ramin, Malcolm Reid, Nikolaos I. Rousis, Yeonsuk Ryu, Pim de Voogt, Jorgen Bramness, and Kevin Thomas, "Comparison of Pharmaceutical, Illicit Drug, Alcohol, Nicotine and Caffeine Levels in Wastewater with Sale, Seizure and Consumption Data for 8 European Cities," *BMC Public Health*, Vol. 16, No. 1, 2016, p. 1035.

BCCSU—*See* British Columbia Centre on Substance Use.

"B.C.'s Top Doctor Calls for Regulated Opioid Supply After Almost 1,500 Overdose Deaths in 2018," CBC News, February 7, 2019. As of July 11, 2019:
https://www.cbc.ca/news/canada/british-columbia/
bonnie-henry-opioid-deaths-1.5009950

Bonello, Deborah, "The Fentanyl Epidemic's Other Victim: Mexican Poppy Farmers," *The Daily Dose*, March 20, 2019. As of July 11, 2019:
https://www.ozy.com/fast-forward/
the-fentanyl-epidemics-other-victim-mexican-poppy-farmers/93117

Booth, Martin, *Opium: A History*, New York: St. Martin's Griffin, 1996.

Bosio, Elisabetta, Mara Mignone, and Elisa Norio, "The New Deal of Fentanyl: A Comparison Between the U.S. and the European Criminal Markets," in *International Scientific Conference "Archibald Reiss Days" Thematic Conference Proceedings of International Significance*, Belgrade, Serbia, October 2–3, 2018, pp. 329–344.

Boyum, David, "Reflections on Economic Theory and Drug Enforcement," dissertation, Harvard University, 1992.

Bretteville-Jensen, Anne Line, and Matthew Sutton, "The Income-Generating Behaviour of Injecting Drug-Users in Oslo," *Addiction*, Vol. 91, No. 1, 1996, pp. 63–79.

British Columbia Coroners Service, *Illicit Drug Toxicity Deaths in BC: January 1, 2009–May 31, 2019*, British Columbia: Ministry of Public Safety and Solicitor General, 2019. As of July 11, 2019:
https://www2.gov.bc.ca/assets/gov/birth-adoption-death-marriage-and-divorce/
deaths/coroners-service/statistical/illicit-drug.pdf

British Columbia Centre on Substance Use, *Heroin Compassion Clubs: A Cooperative Model to Reduce Opioid Overdose Deaths and Disrupt Organized Crime's Role in Fentanyl, Money Laundering and Housing Unaffordability*, Vancouver, British Columbia, February 2019. As of July 11, 2019:
http://www.bccsu.ca/wp-content/uploads/2019/02/
Report-Heroin-Compassion-Clubs.pdf

Brown, Thomas Kingsley, and Kenneth Alper, "Treatment of Opioid Use Disorder with Ibogaine: Detoxification and Drug Use Outcomes," *American Journal of Drug and Alcohol Abuse*, Vol. 44, No. 1, 2018, pp. 24–36.

Burgard, Daniel A., Jason Williams, Danielle Westerman, Rosie Rushing, Riley Carpenter, Addison LaRock, Jane Sadetsky, Jackson Clarke, Heather Fryhle, Melissa Pellman, and Caleb J. Banta-Green, "Using Wastewater-Based Analysis to Monitor the Effects of Legalized Retail Sales on Cannabis Consumption in Washington State, USA," *Addiction*, Vol. 114, No. 9, 2019, pp. 1582–1590.

Byik, Andre, "Chico Police Release Man's Cause of Death in Apparent Mass Overdose," *Chico Enterprise-Record*, January 30, 2019. As of August 23, 2019:
https://www.chicoer.com/2019/01/30/
chico-police-release-mans-cause-of-death-in-apparent-mass-overdose/

Canadian Centre on Substance Use and Addiction, *CCENDU Drug Alert: Illicit Fentanyl*, Ottawa, Ontario, 2013. As of July 11, 2019:
https://www.ccsa.ca/sites/default/files/2019-05/
CCSA-CCENDU-Drug-Alert-Illicit-Fentanyl-2013-en.pdf

Canadian Centre on Substance Use and Addiction, *CCENDU Drug Alert: Increasing Availability of Counterfeit Oxycodone Tablets Containing Fentanyl*, Ottawa, Ontario, 2014. As of July 11, 2019:
https://www.ccsa.ca/sites/default/files/2019-05/
CCSA-CCENDU-Oxycontin-Fentanyl-Alert-2014-en.pdf

Carroll, Jennifer J., Brandon David Lewis Marshall, Josiah D. Rich, and Traci C. Green, "Exposure to Fentanyl-Contaminated Heroin and Overdose Risk Among Illicit Opioid Users in Rhode Island: A Mixed Methods Study," *International Journal of Drug Policy*, Vol. 46, 2017, pp. 136–145.

Casale, John F., Jennifer R. Mallette, and Elizabeth M. Guest, "Analysis of Illicit Carfentanil: Emergence of the Death Dragon," *Forensic Chemistry*, Vol. 3, 2017, pp. 74–80.

Castiglioni, Sara, ed., *Assessing Illicit Drugs in Wastewater: Advances in Wastewater-Based Drug Epidemiology*, Luxembourg: European Monitoring Centre for Drugs and Drug Addiction, 2016. As of July 11, 2019:
http://www.emcdda.europa.eu/system/files/publications/2273/
TDXD16022ENC_4.pdf

Cauchon, Dennis, "Where Is Fentanyl Added to Cocaine? Mostly in Ohio. Result: 3,000 Dead," Harm Reduction Ohio, January 13, 2019. As of July 11, 2019:
https://www.harmreductionohio.org/
where-is-fentanyl-added-to-cocaine-mostly-in-ohio/

Caulkins, Jonathan P., "The Distribution and Consumption of Illicit Drugs: Some Mathematical Models and Their Policy Implications," dissertation, Massachusetts Institute of Technology, 1990. As of July 23, 2019:
https://dspace.mit.edu/handle/1721.1/14022

Caulkins, Jonathan P., "Models Pertaining to How Drug Policy Should Vary over the Course of an Epidemic Cycle," in Björn Lindgren and Michael Grossman, eds., *Substance Use: Individual Behavior, Social Interactions, Markets, and Politics*, Amsterdam, Netherlands: Elsevier, Vol. 16, 2005, pp. 407–439.

Caulkins, Jonathan P., "Price and Purity Analysis for Illicit Drug: Data and Conceptual Issues," *Drug and Alcohol Dependence*, Vol. 90, 2007, pp. S61–S68.

Caulkins, Jonathan P., Honora Burnett, and Edward Leslie, "How Illegal Drugs Enter an Island Country: Insights from Interviews with Incarcerated Smugglers," *Global Crime*, Vol. 10, No. 1-2, 2009, pp. 66–93.

Caulkins, Jonathan P., Emma Disley, Marina Tzvetkova, Mafalda Pardal, Hemali Shah, and Xiaoke Zhang, "Modeling the Structure and Operation of Drug Supply Chains: The Case of Cocaine and Heroin in Italy and Slovenia," *International Journal of Drug Policy*, Vol. 31, 2016, pp. 64–73.

Caulkins, Jonathan P., Benjamin Gurga, and Christopher Little, "Economic Analysis of Drug Transaction 'Cycles' Described by Incarcerated UK Drug Dealers," *Global Crime*, Vol. 10, No. 1-2, 2009, pp. 94–112.

Caulkins, Jonathan P., Beau Kilmer, Peter H. Reuter, and Greg Midgette, "Cocaine's Fall and Marijuana's Rise: Questions and Insights Based on New Estimates of Consumption and Expenditures in U.S. Drug Markets," *Addiction*, Vol. 110, No. 5, 2015, pp. 728–736.

Caulkins, Jonathan P., Bryce Pardo, and Beau Kilmer, "Supervised Consumption Sites: A Nuanced Assessment of the Causal Evidence," *Addiction*, 2019.

Caulkins, Jonathan P., and Peter Reuter, "The Meaning and Utility of Drug Prices," *Addiction*, Vol. 91, 1996, pp. 1261–1264.

Caulkins, Jonathan P., and Peter Reuter, "What Price Data Tell Us About Drug Markets," *Journal of Drug Issues*, Vol. 28, No. 3, 1998, pp. 593–612.

Caulkins, Jonathan P., and Peter Reuter, "Towards a Harm-Reduction Approach to Enforcement," *Safer Communities*, Vol. 8, No. 1, 2009, pp. 9–23.

Caulkins, Jonathan P., and Peter Reuter, "How Drug Enforcement Affects Drug Prices," *Crime and Justice*, Vol. 39, No. 1, 2010, pp. 213–271.

CBP—*See* U.S. Customs and Border Protection.

CCENDU—*See* Canadian Centre on Substance Use and Addiction.

CDC—*See* Centers for Disease Control and Prevention.

Center for Behavioral Health Statistics and Quality, *2017 National Survey on Drug Use and Health: Methodological Summary and Definitions*, Rockville, Md.: Substance Abuse and Mental Health Services Administration, 2018. As of July 23, 2019:
https://www.samhsa.gov/data/
report/2017-methodological-summary-and-definitions

Centers for Disease Control and Prevention, "Nonpharmaceutical Fentanyl-Related Deaths—Multiple States, April 2005–March 2007," *Morbidity and Mortality Weekly Report*, Vol. 57, No. 29, July 25, 2008. As of July 11, 2019:
https://www.cdc.gov/mmwr/preview/mmwrhtml/mm5729a1.htm

Centers for Disease Control and Prevention, *HIV Surveillance Report*, Vol. 23, Washington, D.C., February 2013. As of July 30, 2019:
https://www.cdc.gov/hiv/pdf/
statistics_2011_HIV_Surveillance_Report_vol_23.pdf

Centers for Disease Control and Prevention, "Bridged-Race Resident Population Estimates United States, State and County for the Years 1990–2018," database, June 25, 2019. As of July 11, 2019:
https://wonder.cdc.gov/wonder/help/bridged-race.html

Central Statistical Bureau of Latvia, "ISG010: Population, Population Change, and Key Vital Statistics," data set, 2019. As of July 23, 2019:
http://data1.csb.gov.lv/pxweb/en/iedz/iedz__iedzskaits__ikgad/ISG010.px

Centre for Global Public Health, *Estimation of Key Population Size of People Who Use Injection Drugs (PWID), Men Who Have Sex with Men (MSM) and Sex Workers (SW) Who Are at Risk of Acquiring HIV and Hepatitis C in the Five Health Regions of the Province of British Columbia*, Winnipeg, Manitoba: University of Manitoba, October 5, 2016. As of July 11, 2019:
http://www.bccdc.ca/resource-gallery/Documents/Statistics%20and%20Research/Statistics%20and%20Reports/STI/PSE%20Project%20Final%20Report.pdf

Christie, Chris, Charlie Baker, Roy Cooper, Patrick J. Kennedy, Bertha Madras, and Pam Bondi, *The President's Commission on Combating Drug Addiction and the Opioid Crisis*, Washington, D.C.: U.S. Government Printing Office, November 1, 2017. As of July 11, 2019:
https://www.whitehouse.gov/sites/whitehouse.gov/files/images/Final_Report_Draft_11-1-2017.pdf

Ciccarone, Daniel, "Heroin in Brown, Black and White: Structural Factors and Medical Consequences in the U.S. Heroin Market," *International Journal of Drug Policy*, Vol. 20, No. 3, 2009, pp. 277–282.

Ciccarone, Daniel, "Fentanyl in the U.S. Heroin Supply: A Rapidly Changing Risk Environment," *International Journal of Drug Policy*, Vol. 46, 2017, pp. 107–111.

Ciccarone, Daniel, Jeff Ondocsin, and Sarah G. Mars, "Heroin Uncertainties: Exploring Users' Perceptions of Fentanyl-Adulterated and -Substituted 'Heroin,'" *International Journal on Drug Policy*, Vol. 46, 2017, pp. 146–155.

Cicero, Theodore J., Matthew S. Ellis, and Hilary L. Surratt, "Effect of Abuse-Deterrent Formulation of OxyContin," *New England Journal of Medicine*, Vol. 367, No. 2, 2012, pp. 187–189.

Code of Federal Regulations 21, Part 1310, Control of a Chemical Precursor Used in the Illicit Manufacture of Fentanyl as a List I Chemical: Interim Rule with Request for Comments, Drug Enforcement Administration, U.S. Department of Justice, 2007. As of July 11, 2019:
https://www.deadiversion.usdoj.gov/fed_regs/rules/2007/fr0423.htm

Code of Federal Regulations 21, Part 1310, Control of a Chemical Precursor Used in the Illicit Manufacture of Fentanyl as a List I Chemical: Final Rule, Drug Enforcement Administration, U.S. Department of Justice, 2008. As of July 11, 2019:
https://www.deadiversion.usdoj.gov/fed_regs/rules/2008/fr0725.htm

Coleman, John J., *Fentanyl Analogs in Street Drugs*, Fairfax, Va.: Prescription Drug Research Center, 2007.

"Committee Approves Bill Decriminalizing Drug," Associated Press, March 25, 2019. As of July 23, 2019:
https://www.apnews.com/bc4f3b5880f347a58c29abf2f1b1ee97

Courtwright, David T., *Forces of Habit: Drugs and the Making of the Modern World*, Cambridge, Mass.: Harvard University Press, 2009.

Crenshaw, Zach, "Valley Crime Lab Seeing an Escalation of Fentanyl in Drugs," KNXV Phoenix Metro News, May 24, 2019. As of July 11, 2019:
https://www.abc15.com/news/region-phoenix-metro/
valley-crime-lab-seeing-an-escalation-of-fentanyl-in-street-drugs

Crosby, Michael, Pradan Pattanayak, Sanjeev Verma, and Vignesh Kalyanaraman, "Blockchain Technology: Beyond Bitcoin," *Applied Innovation Review*, Vol. 2, June 2016, pp. 6–20.

Daly, Max, "The Truth About Drug Dealers Lacing Cocaine with Fentanyl," *Vice*, April 5, 2019. As of July 11, 2019:
https://www.vice.com/en_us/article/8xyzkp/
the-truth-about-drug-dealers-lacing-cocaine-with-fentanyl

Daniulaityte, Raminta, Matthew P. Juhascik, Kraig E. Strayer, Ioana E. Sizemore, Kent E. Harshbarger, Heather M. Antonides, and Robert R. Carlson, "Overdose Deaths Related to Fentanyl and Its Analogs—Ohio, January–February 2017," *Morbidity and Mortality Weekly Report*, Vol. 66, No. 34, 2017, pp. 904–908.

DEA—*See* U.S. Drug Enforcement Administration.

DEA NFLIS—*See* U.S. Drug Enforcement Administration, National Forensic Laboratory Information System.

Debruyne, Arthur, "An Invisible Fentanyl Crisis Is Emerging on Mexico's Northern Border," *Pacific Standard*, February 6, 2019. As of July 11, 2019:
https://psmag.com/social-justice/a-fentanyl-epidemic-is-rising-in-northern-mexico

Demaret, Isabelle, Etienne Quertemont, Géraldine Litran, Cécile Magoga, Clémence Deblire, Nathalie Dubois, Jérôme De Roubaix, Corinne Charlier, André Lemaître, Marc Ansseau, "Efficacy of Heroin-Assisted Treatment in Belgium: A Randomised Controlled Trial," *European Addiction Research*, Vol. 21, No. 4, 2015, pp. 179–187.

Denissov, Gleb, *Drug Overdose Mortality in Estonia*, Tallinn, Estonia: National Institute for Health Development, October 16, 2014. As of July 23, 2019: http://www.emcdda.europa.eu/attachements.cfm/att_232697_EN_1.%20G.%20 Denissov%20-%20Drug%20Overdose%20Mortality%20in%20Estonia.pdf

Desroches, Frederick, "Research on Upper Level Drug Trafficking: A Review," *Journal of Drug Issues*, Vol. 37, No. 4, 2007, pp. 827–844.

Dorn, Nicholas, Leslie King, Melanie Defruytier, Freya Van der Laenen, Nacer Lalam, Lorenz Boellinger, Paola Monzini, Isabel Germán, and Xabier Arana, *Literature Review on Upper Level Drug Trafficking*, London: Home Office, 2005.

Eddy, Nathan B., "The History of the Development of Narcotics," *Law and Contemporary Problems*, Vol. 22, No. 1, 1957, pp. 3–8.

Eibl, Joseph K., Kristen Morin, Esa Leinonen, and David C. Marsh, "The State of Opioid Agonist Therapy in Canada 20 Years After Federal Oversight," *Canadian Journal of Psychiatry*, Vol. 62, No. 7, 2017, pp. 444–450.

EMCDDA—*See* European Monitoring Centre for Drugs and Drug Addiction.

Estonian Cause of Death Registry, "RV0211: Mean Annual Population by Sex and Age Group," data set, 2019. As of July 23, 2019: http://andmebaas.stat.ee/Index.aspx?DataSetCode=RV0211

European Monitoring Centre for Drugs and Drug Addiction, *Drug Policy Profiles: Portugal*, Luxembourg: Publications Office of the European Union, 2011. As of July 11, 2019: http://www.emcdda.europa.eu/publications/drug-policy-profiles/portugal_en

European Monitoring Centre for Drugs and Drug Addiction, *Sweden: Country Drug Report 2017*, Luxembourg: Publications Office of the European Union, 2017. As of July 11, 2019: http://www.emcdda.europa.eu/publications/country-drug-reports/2017/sweden_en

European Monitoring Centre for Drugs and Drug Addiction, *Estonia: Country Drug Report 2018*, Luxembourg: Publications Office of the European Union, 2018a. As of July 11, 2019: http://www.emcdda.europa.eu/publications/country-drug-reports/2018/estonia_en

European Monitoring Centre for Drugs and Drug Addiction, *European Drug Report 2018: Trends and Developments*, Luxembourg: Publications Office of the European Union, 2018b. As of July 11, 2019: http://www.emcdda.europa.eu/publications/edr/trends-developments/2018_en

European Monitoring Centre for Drugs and Drug Addiction, *Finland: Country Drug Report 2018*, Luxembourg: Publications Office of the European Union, 2018c. As of July 11, 2019: http://www.emcdda.europa.eu/system/files/publications/11303/ finland-cdr-2018-with-numbers.pdf

European Monitoring Centre for Drugs and Drug Addiction, *Latvia: Country Drug Report 2018*, Luxembourg: Publications Office of the European Union, 2018d. As of July 11, 2019:
http://www.emcdda.europa.eu/publications/country-drug-reports/2018/latvia_en

European Monitoring Centre for Drugs and Drug Addiction, *Lithuania: Country Drug Report 2018*, Luxembourg: Publications Office of the European Union, 2018e. As of July 11, 2019:
http://www.emcdda.europa.eu/publications/country-drug-reports/2018/lithuania_en

European Monitoring Centre for Drugs and Drug Addiction, *Sweden: Country Drug Report 2018*, Luxembourg: Publications Office of the European Union, 2018f. As of July 11, 2019:
http://www.emcdda.europa.eu/publications/country-drug-reports/2018/sweden_en

European Monitoring Centre for Drugs and Drug Addiction, *Estonia: Country Drug Report 2019*, Luxembourg: Publications Office of the European Union, 2019a. As of July 11, 2019:
http://www.emcdda.europa.eu/publications/country-drug-reports/2019/estonia_en

European Monitoring Centre for Drugs and Drug Addiction, *Finland: Country Drug Report 2019*, Luxembourg: Publications Office of the European Union, 2019b. As of July 11, 2019:
http://www.emcdda.europa.eu/publications/country-drug-reports/2019/finland_en

European Monitoring Centre for Drugs and Drug Addiction, *Latvia: Country Drug Report 2019*, Luxembourg: Publications Office of the European Union, 2019c. As of July 11, 2019:
http://www.emcdda.europa.eu/publications/country-drug-reports/2019/latvia_en

European Monitoring Centre for Drugs and Drug Addiction, *Perspectives on Drugs—Wastewater Analysis and Drugs: A European Multi-City Study*, Luxembourg: Publications Office of the European Union, 2019d. As of July 11, 2019:
http://www.emcdda.europa.eu/publications/pods/waste-water-analysis_en

European Monitoring Centre for Drugs and Drug Addiction, "Statistical Bulletin 2019—Overdose Deaths," webpage, 2019e. As of July 11, 2019:
http://www.emcdda.europa.eu/data/stats2019/drd

European Monitoring Centre for Drugs and Drug Addiction, *Sweden: Country Drug Report 2019*, Luxembourg: Publications Office of the European Union, 2019f. As of July 11, 2019:
http://www.emcdda.europa.eu/publications/country-drug-reports/2019/sweden_en

European Monitoring Centre for Drugs and Drug Addiction, *Drug-Related Deaths and Mortality in Europe: Update from the EMCDDA Expert Network*, Luxembourg: Publications Office of the European Union, July 2019g. As of August 2, 2019:
http://www.emcdda.europa.eu/system/files/publications/11485/
20193286_TD0319444ENN_PDF.pdf

Europol, *Amphetamine-Type Stimulants in the European Union 1998–2007: Europol Contribution to the Expert Consultations for the UNGASS Assessment*, The Hague, Netherlands, July 2007. As of July 11, 2019:
http://edz.bib.uni-mannheim.de/daten/edz-min/pol/04/
EuropolUNGASSAssessment.pdf

Europol, *Internet Organised Crime Threat Assessment*, The Hague, Netherlands: European Cybercrime Centre, 2018. As of July 23, 2019:
https://www.europol.europa.eu/internet-organised-crime-threat-assessment-2018

Evans-Brown, Michael, Ana Gallegos, Rachel Christie, Sofía Sola, Anabela Almeida, Rita Jorge, Joanna De Morais, and Roumen Sedefov, *Fentanils and Synthetic Cannabinoids: Driving Greater Complexity into the Drug Situation—An Update from the EU Early Warning-System*, Luxembourg: Publications Office of the European Union, June 2018. As of July 11, 2019:
http://www.emcdda.europa.eu/system/files/publications/8870/
2018-2489-td0118414enn.pdf

Everingham, Susan M., C. Peter Rydell, and Jonathan P. Caulkins, "Cocaine Consumption in the United States: Estimating Past Trends and Future Scenarios," *Socio-Economic Planning Sciences*, Vol. 29, No. 4, 1995, pp. 305–314.

"Fentanyl Found for the First Time in Illegal Quebec Drug Lab, Says SQ," CBC News, December 27, 2016. As of July 11, 2019:
https://www.cbc.ca/news/canada/montreal/
fentanyl-found-quebec-drug-lab-bust-sq-1.3913621

Ferri, Marica, Marina Davoli, and Carlo A. Perucci, "Heroin Maintenance for Chronic Heroin-Dependent Individuals," *Cochrane Database of Systematic Reviews*, Vol. 7, No. 12, December 2011.

Finnish National Focal Point, *Finland: Drug Situation 2003*, Helsinki, Finland, 2004.

Finnish National Focal Point, *Finland: Drug Situation 2005—New Developments, Trends, and In-Depth Information on Selected Issues*, Helsinki, Finland, 2006. As of July 11, 2019:
http://www.emcdda.europa.eu/attachements.cfm/
att_34591_EN_NR2005Finland.pdf

Firestone, Michelle, Brian Goldman, and Benedikt Fischer, "Fentanyl Use Among Street Drug Users in Toronto, Canada: Behavioural Dynamics and Public Health Implications," *International Journal of Drug Policy*, Vol. 20, No. 1, 2009, pp. 90–92.

Fischer, Benedikt, Cayley Russell, Yoko Murphy, and Paul Kurdyak, "Prescription Opioids, Abuse and Public Health in Canada: Is Fentanyl the New Centre of the Opioid Crisis?" *Pharmacoepidemiology and Drug Safety*, Vol. 24, No. 12, 2015, pp. 1334–1336.

Fischer, Benedikt, Thepikaa Varatharajan, Kevin Shield, Jürgen Rehm, and Wayne Jones, "Crude Estimates of Prescription Opioid-Related Misuse and Use Disorder Populations Towards Informing Intervention System Need in Canada," *Drug and Alcohol Dependence*, Vol. 189, 2018, pp. 76–79.

Fischer, Benedikt, Lenka Vojtila, and Jürgen Rehm, "The 'Fentanyl Epidemic' in Canada–Some Cautionary Observations Focusing on Opioid-Related Mortality," *Preventive Medicine*, Vol. 107, 2018, pp. 109–113.

Forman, Robert F., "Availability of Opioids on the Internet," *JAMA*, Vol. 290, No. 7, 2003, p. 889.

Forssell, Marta, and Tuula Nurmi, *Päihdehuollon huumeasiakkaat 2013*, National Institute for Health and Welfare, 2014.

Freeborn, Beth A., "Arrest Avoidance: Law Enforcement and the Price of Cocaine," *Journal of Law and Economics*, Vol. 52, No. 1, 2009, pp. 19–40.

Fu Jun-ke, Ren Li-jun, Xiang Yu-lian, Fan Qi-ping, and Tian Xing-Tao, "A Developed Method for Synthesis of Fentanyl," *Chinese Journal of Medicinal Chemistry*, 2011.

Fugelstad, Anna, "Large Increase in Opioid-Related Deaths in Sweden," Karolinska Institutet, briefing, 2015. As of July 11, 2019:
https://www.med.uio.no/klinmed/forskning/sentre/seraf/aktuelt/arrangementer/konferanser/konferanser-2015/overdosekonferansen-2015/fugelstad---large-increace-in-opioid-related-death-in-sweden.pdf

Galenianos, Manolis, Rosalie Liccardo Pacula, and Nicola Persico, "A Search-Theoretic Model of the Retail Market for Illicit Drugs," *Review of Economic Studies*, Vol. 79, No. 3, 2012, pp. 1239–1269.

Gallet, Craig A. "Can Price Get the Monkey off Our Back? A Meta-Analysis of Illicit Drug Demand," *Health Economics*, Vol. 23, No. 1, 2014, pp. 55–68.

Ghaffarzadeh, Mohammad, Somaye Shahrivari Joghan, and Fereshteh Faraji, "A New Method for the Synthesis of Amides from Imines," *Tetrahedron Letters*, Vol. 53, No. 2, 2012, pp. 203–206.

Gilbert, Michael, and Nabarun Dasgupta, "Silicon to Syringe: Cryptomarkets and Disruptive Innovation in Opioid Supply Chains," *International Journal of Drug Policy*, Vol. 46, 2017, pp. 160–167.

Gill, Hannah, Eamonn Kelly, and Graeme Henderson, "How the Complex Pharmacology of the Fentanyls Contributes to Their Lethality," *Addiction*, Vol. 114, No. 9, 2019, pp. 1524–1525.

Gladden, R. Matthew, Pedro Martinez, and Puja Seth, "Fentanyl Law Enforcement Submissions and Increases in Synthetic Opioid-Involved Overdose Deaths—27 States, 2013–2014," *Morbidity and Mortality Weekly Report*, Vol. 65, No. 33, 2016, pp. 837–843.

Gomes, Tara, Wayne Khuu, Diana Martins, Mina Tadrous, Muhammad M. Mamdani, J. Michael Paterson, and David N. Juurlink, "Contributions of Prescribed and Non-Prescribed Opioids to Opioid Related Deaths: Population Based Cohort Study in Ontario, Canada," *BMJ*, Vol. 362, 2018.

Grandmaison, Romain Le Cour, Nathaniel Morris, and Benjamin T. Smith, *The U.S. Fentanyl Boom and the Mexican Opium Crisis: Finding Opportunities Amidst Violence?* Washington, D.C.: Wilson Center and Network of Researchers in International Affairs, February 2019. As of July 11, 2019: https://www.wilsoncenter.org/sites/default/files/ the_u.s._fentanyl_boom_and_the_mexican_opium_crisis.pdf

Greenfield, Victoria A., and Letizia Paoli, "If Supply-Oriented Drug Policy Is Broken, Can Harm Reduction Help Fix it? Melding Disciplines and Methods to Advance International Drug-Control Policy," *International Journal of Drug Policy*, Vol. 23, No. 1, 2012, pp. 6–15.

Gribova, A., *Drug Markets and Crime Workbook 2018: Latvia*, Riga, Latvia, 2018. Not available to the general public.

Guerrero Castro, Javier Enrique, "Maritime Interdiction in the War on Drugs in Colombia: Practices, Technologies and Technological Innovation," *Small Wars Journal*, July 7, 2017. As of July 11, 2019: https://smallwarsjournal.com/blog/maritime-interdiction-in-the-war-on-drugs-in- colombia-practices-technologies-and-technological-

Gunnar, Teemu, and Aino Kankaanpää, "Jätevesitutkimus," National Institute for Health and Welfare, webpage, 2018. As of July 11, 2019: https://thl.fi/fi/tutkimus-ja-kehittaminen/tutkimukset-ja-hankkeet/ jatevesitutkimus

Gunnar, T., A. Kankaanpää, K. Karjalainen, and S. Ronka, *Drugs Workbook 2018: Finland*, Helsinki, Finland, 2018. Not available to the general public.

Gupta, Pradeep Kumar, Kumaran Ganesan, Ambuja Pande, and Ramesh Chandra Malhotra, "A Convenient One-Pot Synthesis of Fentanyl," *Journal of Chemical Research*, Vol. 36, 2005, pp. 452–453.

Gupta, Pradeep Kumar, Shiv Kumar Yadav, Yangchen Doma Bhutia, Poonam Singh, Pooja Rao, Niranjan Laxman Gujar, Kumaran Ganesan, Rahul Bhattacharya, "Synthesis and Comparative Bioefficacy of *N*-(1-phenethyl-4-piperidinyl) Propionanilide (Fentanyl) and Its 1-Substituted Analogs in Swiss Albino Mice," *Medicinal Chemistry Research*, Vol. 22, No. 8, 2013, pp. 3888–3896.

Guthrie, Amy, "Mexican Poppy Producing State Pushes to Decriminalize Opium," Associated Press, August 19, 2018. As of July 11, 2019:
https://www.apnews.com/4c263918b589454c8b1c46c8bfcb45f5

Haasen, Christian, Uwe Verthein, Peter Degkwitz, Juergen Berger, Michael Krausz, and Dieter Naber, "Heroin-Assisted Treatment for Opioid Dependence: Randomised Controlled Trial," British Journal of Psychiatry, Vol. 191, No. 1, 2007, pp. 55–62.

Hamilton, Keegan, "How the Sinaloa Cartel Is Using Chinese Chemicals to Fuel America's Opioid Crisis," Vice News, January 12, 2019. As of July 11, 2019:
https://www.vice.com/en_asia/article/pa5nbk/
how-the-sinaloa-cartel-is-using-chinese-chemicals-to-fuel-americas-opioid-crisis

Harm Reduction Coalition, "DOPE Project: Case Study," webpage, undated. As of July 11, 2019:
https://harmreduction.org/issues/overdose-prevention/tools-best-practices/
naloxone-program-case-studies/dope-project/

Hayashi, Kanna, M-J Milloy, Mark Lysyshyn, Kora DeBeck, Ekaterina Nosova, Evan Wood, and Thomas Kerr, "Substance Use Patterns Associated with Recent Exposure to Fentanyl Among People Who Inject Drugs in Vancouver, Canada: A Cross-Sectional Urine Toxicology Screening Study," Drug and Alcohol Dependence, Vol. 183, 2018, pp. 1–6.

Health Canada, "Methadone Program," webpage, updated April 27, 2017. As of July 11, 2019:
https://www.canada.ca/en/health-canada/services/health-concerns/
controlled-substances-precursor-chemicals/exemptions/methadone-program.html

Health Canada, "Supervised Consumption Sites: Status of Applications," webpage, updated July 19, 2019. As of July 19, 2019:
https://www.canada.ca/en/health-canada/services/substance-use/
supervised-consumption-sites/status-application.html

Health Canada, Drug Analysis Service, "Summary Report of Samples Analyzed 2016," data set, December 1, 2017. As of July 23, 2019:
https://www.canada.ca/en/health-canada/services/health-concerns/
controlled-substances-precursor-chemicals/drug-analysis-service/
2016-drug-analysis-service-summary-report-samples-analysed.html

Health Canada, Drug Analysis Service, "Summary Report of Samples Analyzed 2017," data set, June 26, 2018. As of July 23, 2019:
https://www.canada.ca/en/health-canada/services/health-concerns/
controlled-substances-precursor-chemicals/drug-analysis-service/
2017-drug-analysis-service-summary-report-samples-analysed.html

Health Canada, Drug Analysis Service, "Summary Report of Samples Analyzed 2018," data set, July 17, 2019a. As of July 23, 2019:
https://www.canada.ca/en/health-canada/services/health-concerns/
controlled-substances-precursor-chemicals/drug-analysis-service/
2018-drug-analysis-service-summary-report-samples-analysed.html

Health Canada, Drug Analysis Service, "2019 Analyzed Drug Report—Quarter 1," data set, July 22, 2019b. As of July 23, 2019:
https://www.canada.ca/en/health-canada/services/health-concerns/
controlled-substances-precursor-chemicals/drug-analysis-service/
2019-analyzed-drug-report-q1.html

Hedegaard, Holly, Brigham A. Bastian, James P. Trinidad, Merianne Spencer, and Margaret Warner, "Drugs Most Frequently Involved in Drug Overdose Deaths: United States, 2011–2016," *National Vital Statistics Reports*, Vol. 67, No. 9, December 12, 2018, pp. 1–14.

Hedegaard, Holly, Arialdi M. Miniño, and Margaret Warner, *Drug Overdose Deaths in the United States, 1999–2017*, Hyattsville, Md.: National Center for Health Statistics, Centers for Disease Control and Prevention, Data Brief No. 329, November 2018. As of July 11, 2019:
https://www.cdc.gov/nchs/data/databriefs/db329-h.pdf

Hempstead, Katherine, and Emel O. Yildirim, "Supply-Side Response to Declining Heroin Purity: Fentanyl Overdose Episode in New Jersey," *Health Economics*, Vol. 23, No. 6, 2014, pp. 688–705.

Henderson, G. L., "Designer Drugs: Past History and Future Prospects," *Journal of Forensic Science*, Vol. 33, No. 2, 1988, pp. 569–575.

Hermanson, Terhi, and Pekka Järvinen, "Schengen Bans the Purchase of Buprenorphine from France: Drug Transport Between Schengen Countries Requires a Pharmacy Certificate," *Lääkärilehti Medical Journal*, 2003, pp. 549–551.

Hibbs, Jonathan, Joshua Perper, and Charles L. Winek, "An Outbreak of Designer Drug-Related Deaths in Pennsylvania," *JAMA*, Vol. 265, No. 8, 1991, pp. 1011–1013.

Ho, Joel, Kora DeBeck, M-J Milloy, Huiru Dong, Evan Wood, Thomas Kerr, and Kanna Hayashi, "Increasing Availability of Illicit and Prescription Opioids Among People Who Inject Drugs in a Canadian Setting, 2010–2014," *American Journal of Drug and Alcohol Abuse*, Vol. 44, No. 3, 2018, pp. 368–377.

Hrymak, Haley, "The Opioid Crisis as Health Crisis, Not Criminal Crisis: Implications for the Criminal Justice System," thesis, University of British Columbia, 2018. As of July 11, 2019:
https://open.library.ubc.ca/cIRcle/collections/ubctheses/24/items/1.0371246

Hsu, Fu-Lian, and Harold D. Banks, *Fentanyl Synthetic Methodology: A Comparative Study*, Aberdeen Proving Ground, Md.: U.S. Army Armament Munitions Chemical Command, 1992.

Hughes, Caitlin Elizabeth, and Alex Stevens, "What Can We Learn from the Portuguese Decriminalization of Illicit Drugs?" *British Journal of Criminology*, Vol. 50, No. 6, 2010, pp. 999–1022.

Humphreys, Keith, Jonathan P. Caulkins, and Vanda Felbab-Brown, "Opioids of the Masses: Stopping an American Epidemic from Going Global," *Foreign Affairs*, Vol. 97, 2018. As of July 11, 2019:
https://www.foreignaffairs.com/articles/world/2018-04-16/opioids-masses

International Narcotics Control Board, "INCB: Scheduling of Fentanyl Precursors Comes into Force," press release, October 18, 2017. As of July 11, 2019:
https://www.incb.org/incb/en/news/press-releases/2017/
press_release_20171018.html

International Narcotics Control Board, *Narcotic Drugs: Estimated World Requirements for 2019: Statistics for 2017*, New York: United Nations, 2019. As of July 11, 2019:
https://www.drugsandalcohol.ie/30398/1/
INCB-Narcotics_Drugs_Technical_Publication_2018.pdf

Iosebashvili, Ira, "Mexican Peso Falls to Lowest Level Against Dollar in over a Year," *Wall Street Journal*, November 26, 2018. As of July 11, 2019:
https://www.wsj.com/articles/
mexican-peso-falls-to-lowest-level-against-dollar-in-over-a-year-1543259849

Irvine, Michael A., Margot Kuo, Jane A. Buxton, Robert Balshaw, Michael Otterstatter, Laura Macdougall, M.-J. Milloy, Aamir Bharmal, Bonnie Henry, Mark Tyndall, Daniel Coombs, and Mark Gilbert, "Modelling the Combined Impact of Interventions in Averting Deaths During a Synthetic-Opioid Overdose Epidemic," *Addiction*, Vol. 114, No. 9, 2019, pp. 1602–1613.

Jackson, Anne, "Partial Agonist," in P. Stolerman, ed., *Encyclopedia of Psychopharmacology*, Heidelberg, Germany: Springer-Verlag Berlin Heidelberg, 2010, pp. 959–960.

Janjua, Naveed Zafar, Nazrul Islam, Margot Kuo, Amanda Yu, Stanley Wong, Zahid A. Butt, Mark Gilbert, Jane Buxton, Nuria Chapinal, Hasina Samji, Mei Chong, Maria Alvarez, Jason Wong, Mark W. Tyndall, and Mel Krajden, "Identifying Injection Drug Use and Estimating Population Size of People Who Inject Drugs Using Healthcare Administrative Datasets," *International Journal of Drug Policy*, Vol. 55, 2018, pp. 31–39.

Janssen, Paul A., "Pirinitramide (R 3365), a Potent Analgesic with Unusual Chemical Structure," *Journal of Pharmacy and Pharmacology*, Vol. 13, No. 1, 1961, pp. 513–530.

Janssen, Paul A., and Nathan B. Eddy, "Compounds Related to Pethidine-IV. New General Chemical Methods of Increasing the Analgesic Activity of Pethidine," *Journal of Medicinal and Pharmaceutical Chemistry*, Vol. 2, 1960, pp. 31–45.

Jemal, A., R. Siegel, J. Xu, and E. Ward, "Cancer Statistics, 2010," *CA: A Cancer Journal for Clinicians*, Vol. 60, No. 5, 2010, pp. 277–300.

Johnson, B. D., P. J. Goldstein, E. Preble, J. Schmeidler, D. S. Lipton, B. Spunt, and T. Miller, *Taking Care of Business: The Economics of Crime by Heroin Abusers*, New York: Lexington Books, 1985.

Jonczyk, A., M. Jawdosiuk, M. Makosza, and J. Czyzewski, "Search for a New Method for Synthesis of the Analgesic Agent 'Fentanyl,'" *Chemischer Informationsdienst*, Vol. 9, No. 28, 1978, pp. 131–134.

Jones, Andrea A., Kerry Jang, William J. Panenka, Alasdair M. Barr, G. William MacEwan, Allen E. Thornton, and William G. Honer, "Rapid Change in Fentanyl Prevalence in a Community-Based, High-Risk Sample," *JAMA Psychiatry*, Vol. 75, No. 3, 2018, pp. 298–300.

Kankaanpää, Aino, Kari Ariniemi, Mari Heinonen, Kimmo Kuoppasalmi, and Teemu Gunnar, "Current Trends in Finnish Drug Abuse: Wastewater Based Epidemiology Combined with Other National Indicators," *Science of the Total Environment*, Vol. 568, 2016, pp. 864–874.

Karamouzian, Mohammad, Carolyn Dohoo, Sara Forsting, Ryan McNeil, Thomas Kerr, and Mark Lysyshyn, "Evaluation of a Fentanyl Drug Checking Service for Clients of a Supervised Injection Facility, Vancouver, Canada," *Harm Reduction Journal*, Vol. 15, No. 1, 2018.

Katselou, Maria, Ioannis Papoutsis, Panagiota Nikolaou, Chara Spiliopoulou, and Sotiris Athanaselis, "AH-7921: The List of New Psychoactive Opioids Is Expanded," *Forensic Toxicology*, Vol. 33, No. 2, 2015, pp. 195–201.

Kilmer, Beau, and Jonathan Caulkins, "Hard Drugs Demand Solid Understanding," *USA Today*, March 8, 2014. As of July 11, 2019: https://www.usatoday.com/story/opinion/2014/03/08/heroin-abuse-hoffman-research-column/6134337/

Kilmer, Beau, Jonathan P. Caulkins, Brittany M. Bond, and Peter Reuter, *Reducing Drug Trafficking Revenues and Violence in Mexico: Would Legalizing Marijuana in California Help?* Santa Monica, Calif.: RAND Corporation, OP-325-RC, 2010. As of July 11, 2019: https://www.rand.org/pubs/occasional_papers/OP325.html

Kilmer, Beau, and Robert MacCoun, "Should California Drop Criminal Penalties for Drug Possession?" *San Francisco Chronicle*, July 20, 2017. As of July 11, 2019: https://www.sfchronicle.com/opinion/article/Should-California-drop-criminal-penalties-for-11303420.php

Kilmer, Beau, and Bryce Pardo, "Addressing Federal Conflicts over Supervised Drug Consumption Sites," *The Hill*, March 14, 2019. As of July 11, 2019: https://thehill.com/blogs/congress-blog/healthcare/434045-addressing-federal-conflicts-over-supervised-drug-consumption

Kilmer, Beau, Peter Reuter, and Luca Giommoni, "What Can Be Learned from Cross-National Comparisons of Data on Illegal Drugs?" *Crime and Justice*, Vol. 44, No. 1, 2015, pp. 227–296.

Kilmer, Beau, Rosanna Smart, Jirka Taylor, and Jonathan P. Caulkins, "Prescribing Diamorphine in the United States: Insights from a Nationally Representative Survey," *Drug and Alcohol Dependence*, Vol. 196, 2019, pp. 62–65.

Kilmer, Beau, Jirka Taylor, Jonathan P. Caulkins, Pam A. Mueller, Allison J. Ober, Bryce Pardo, Rosanna Smart, Lucy Strang, and Peter Reuter, *Considering Heroin-Assisted Treatment and Supervised Drug Consumption Sites in the United States*, Santa Monica, Calif.: RAND Corporation, RR-2693-RC, 2018. As of July 11, 2019: https://www.rand.org/pubs/research_reports/RR2693.html

Kleiman, Mark A. R., *Marijuana: Costs of Abuse, Costs of Control*, New York: Greenwood Press, 1989.

Kleiman, Mark, "Opting for Ignorance: ADAM Program Killed," *Same Facts.com*, January 21, 2004. As of July 11, 2019: http://www.samefacts.com/2004/01/drug-policy/opting-for-ignorance-adam-program-killed/

Kleiman, Mark A. R., *When Brute Force Fails: How to Have Less Crime and Less Punishment*, Princeton, N.J.: Princeton University Press, 2009.

Kleiman, Mark, "Surgical Strikes in the Drug Wars: Smarter Policies for Both Sides of the Border," *Foreign Affairs*, Vol. 90, No. 5, 2011, pp. 89–101.

Koenig, Xaver, and Karlheinz Hilber, "The Anti-Addiction Drug Ibogaine and the Heart: A Delicate Relation," *Molecules*, Vol. 20, No. 2, 2015, pp. 2208–2228.

Kramer, C., and M. Tawney, "A Fatal Overdose of Transdermally Administered Fentanyl," *Journal of the American Osteopathic Association*, Vol. 98, No. 7, 1998, pp. 385–386.

Krieger, Maxwell S., Jesse L. Yedinak, Jane A. Buxton, Mark Lysyshyn, Edward Bernstein, Josiah D. Rich, Traci C. Green, Scott E. Hadland, and Brandon D. L. Marshall, "High Willingness to Use Rapid Fentanyl Test Strips Among Young Adults Who Use Drugs," *Harm Reduction Journal*, Vol. 15, No. 7, 2018.

Krikku, P., and S. Ronka, *Harms and Harm Reduction Workbook 2018: Finland*, Helsinki, Finland, 2018. Not available to the general public.

Kronstrand, Robert, Henrik Druid, Per Holmgren, and Jovan Rajs, "A Cluster of Fentanyl-Related Deaths Among Drug Addicts in Sweden," *Forensic Science International*, Vol. 88, No. 3, 1997, pp. 185–195.

Kruithof, Kristy, Judith Aldridge, David Décary-Hétu, Megan Sim, Elma Dujso, and Stijn Hoorens, *Internet-Facilitated Drugs Trade: An Analysis of the Size, Scope and the Role of the Netherlands*, Santa Monica, Calif.: RAND Corporation, RR-1607-WODC, 2016. As of July 11, 2019: https://www.rand.org/pubs/research_reports/RR1607.html

Kund, Oliver, "Historical Moment: Fentanyl Business Halted—Estonian News," *Postimees*, December 6, 2017. As of July 11, 2019: https://news.postimees.ee/4336097/historical-moment-fentanyl-business-halted

Laqueur, Hannah, "Uses and Abuses of Drug Decriminalization in Portugal," *Law and Social Inquiry*, Vol. 40, No. 3, 2015, pp. 746–781.

Legislative Assembly of British Columbia, Bill 27–2018: Pill Press and Related Equipment Control Act, May 10, 2018. As of July 11, 2019: https://www.leg.bc.ca/parliamentary-business/ legislation-debates-proceedings/41st-parliament/3rd-session/bills/ third-reading/gov27-3

Leifman, Håkan, *Drug-Related Deaths—The Swedish Case*, Stockholm, Sweden: CAN, 2016a. As of July 11, 2019: http://www.emcdda.europa.eu/system/files/attachments/3238/ Hakan%20Leifman.pdf

Leifman, Håkan, *Drug-Related Deaths in Sweden—Estimations of Trends, Effects of Changes in Recording Practices and Studies of Drug Patterns*, Stockholm, Sweden: CAN, 2016b. As of July 11, 2019: http://www.emcdda.europa.eu/document-library/drug-related-deaths-sweden-%E2%80%93-estimations-trends-effects-changes-recording-practices-and-studies-drug-patterns_en

Leskinen, J., *Drug Market and Crime Workbook 2018: Finland*, Helsinki, Finland, 2018. Not available to the general public.

Liu Yuejin, "SCIO Briefing on Fentanyl-Related Substances Control," webpage, April 2, 2019. As of July 19, 2019: http://www.china.org.cn/china/2019-04/02/content_74637197.htm

Lombardo, Joseph, and Keith Carter, *Nevada High Intensity Drug Trafficking Area: 2018 Threat Assessment*, Office of National Drug Control Policy, June 15, 2018. As of July 11, 2019: http://casatondemand.org/wp-content/uploads/2018/10/ 2018-nv-hidta-threat-assessment_final-1.pdf

Lopez, German, "Elizabeth Warren's $100 Billion Plan to Fight the Opioid Epidemic, Explained," *Vox*, May 8, 2019. As of July 11, 2019: https://www.vox.com/future-perfect/2019/5/8/18535959/ elizabeth-warren-opioid-epidemic-2020-democratic-campaigns-trump

López-Muñoz, Francisco, and Cecilio Alamo, "The Consolidation of Neuroleptic Therapy: Janssen, the Discovery of Haloperidol and its Introduction into Clinical Practice," *Brain Research Bulletin*, Vol. 79, No. 2, 2009, pp. 130–141.

Lupick, Travis, "Why California Has Largely Been Spared Fentanyl Deaths—So Far," *Filter*, October 2, 2018. As of July 11, 2019: https://filtermag.org/2018/10/02/why-california-has-largely-been-spared-fentanyl-related-deaths-and-the-fight-to-keep-it-that-way/

Lurie, Ira S., Arthur L. Berrier, John F. Casale, Reiko Iio, and Joseph S. Bozenko, Jr., "Profiling of Illicit Fentanyl Using UHPLC–MS/MS," *Forensic Science International*, Vol. 220, No. 1-3, 2012, pp. 191–196.

MacCoun, Robert J., "Testing Drugs Versus Testing for Drug Use: Private Risk Management in the Shadow of Criminal Law," *DePaul Law Review*, Vol. 56, 2006, pp. 507–538.

MacCoun, Robert, and Peter Reuter, "Are the Wages of Sin $30 an Hour? Economic Aspects of Street-Level Drug Dealing," *Crime & Delinquency*, Vol. 38, No. 4, 1992, pp. 477–491.

Mahony, Edmund, "Stalking a 'Serial Killer' Narcotic from Boston to Wichita," *Hartford Courant*, February 23, 1993. As of July 11, 2019: https://www.courant.com/news/connecticut/hc-xpm-1993-02-23-0000105550-story.html

Malaquin, Sandra, Mouhamad Jida, Jean-Claude Gesquiere, Rebecca Deprez-Poulain, Benoit Deprez, and Guillaume Laconde, "Ugi Reaction for the Synthesis of 4-Aminopiperidine-4-Carboxylic Acid Derivatives. Application to the Synthesis of Carfentanil and Remifentanil," *Tetrahedron Letters*, Vol. 51, No. 22, 2010, pp. 2983–2985.

March, Joan Carles, Eugenia Oviedo-Joekes, Emilio Perea-Milla, and Francisco Carrasco, "Controlled Trial of Prescribed Heroin in the Treatment of Opioid Addiction," *Journal of Substance Abuse Treatment*, Vol. 31, No. 2, 2006, pp. 203–211.

Mars, Sarah G., Philippe Bourgois, George Karandinos, Fernando Montero, and Daniel Ciccarone, "'Every "Never" I Ever Said Came True': Transitions from Opioid Pills to Heroin Injecting," *International Journal of Drug Policy*, Vol. 25, No. 2, 2014, pp. 257–266.

Mars, Sarah G., Jeff Ondocsin, and Daniel Ciccarone, "Sold as Heroin: Perceptions and Use of an Evolving Drug in Baltimore, MD," *Journal of Psychoactive Drugs*, Vol. 50, No. 2, 2018a, pp. 167–176.

Mars, Sarah G., Jeff Ondocsin, and Daniel Ciccarone, "Toots, Tastes and Tester Shots: User Accounts of Drug Sampling Methods for Gauging Heroin Potency," *Harm Reduction Journal*, Vol. 15, No. 1, 2018b.

Mars, Sarah G., Daniel Rosenblum, and Daniel Ciccarone, "Illicit Fentanyls in the Opioid Street Market: Desired or Imposed? *Addiction*, Vol. 114, No. 5, 2018, pp. 774–780.

Martin, Eric, and Justin Villamil, "Mexico's Peso Is Expected to Make a Big Comeback," Bloomberg, January 4, 2018. As of July 11, 2019: https://www.bloomberg.com/news/articles/2018-01-04/ mexican-peso-seen-reinvented-as-world-s-best-performing-currency

Martin, James, *Drugs on the Dark Net: How Cryptomarkets Are Transforming the Global Trade in Illicit Drugs*, London: Palgrave Macmillan, 2014.

Martin, Marcus, Janene Hecker, Richard Clark, Jeffrey Frye, Dietrich Jehle, Emily Jean Lucid, and Fred Harchelroad, "China White Epidemic: An Eastern United States Emergency Department Experience," *Annals of Emergency Medicine*, Vol. 20, No. 2, 1991, pp. 158–164.

Mathers, Bradley M., and Louisa Degenhardt, "Examining Non-AIDS Mortality Among People Who Inject Drugs," *AIDS*, Vol. 28, No. 4, 2014, p. S435.

Mattick, R. P., C. Breen, J. Kimber, and M. Davoli, "Methadone Maintenance Therapy Versus No Opioid Replacement Therapy for Opioid Dependence," *Cochrane Database of Systematic Reviews*, Vol. 3, 2009.

Mattick, R. P., C. Breen, J. Kimber, and M. Davoli, "Buprenorphine Maintenance Versus Placebo or Methadone Maintenance for Opioid Dependence," *Cochrane Database of Systematic Reviews*, Vol. 2, February 6, 2014.

Mayer, Brian P., Alan J. DeHope, Daniel A. Mew, Paul E. Spackman, and Audrey M. Williams, "Chemical Attribution of Fentanyl Using Multivariate Statistical Analysis of Orthogonal Mass Spectral Data," *Analytical Chemistry*, Vol. 88, No. 8, 2016.

McGinty, Emma E., Colleen L. Barry, Elizabeth M. Stone, Jeff Niederdeppe, Alene Kennedy-Hendricks, Sarah Linden, and Susan G. Sherman, "Public Support for Safe Consumption Sites and Syringe Services Programs to Combat the Opioid Epidemic," *Preventive Medicine*, Vol. 111, 2018, pp. 73–77.

McKnight, C., and D. C. Des Jarlais, "Being 'Hooked Up' During a Sharp Increase in the Availability of Illicitly Manufactured Fentanyl: Adaptations of Drug Using Practices Among People Who Use Drugs (PWUD) in New York City," *International Journal of Drug Policy*, Vol. 60, 2018, pp. 82–88.

McLellan, A. Thomas, Isabelle O. Arndt, David S. Metzger, George E. Woody, and Charles P. O'Brien, "The Effects of Psychosocial Services in Substance Abuse Treatment," *Addictions Nursing Network*, Vol. 5, No. 2, 1993, pp. 38–47.

McLellan, A. Thomas, Teresa A. Hagan, Marvin Levine, Frank Gould, Kathleen Meyers, Mark Bencivengo, and Jack Durell, "Supplemental Social Services Improve Outcomes in Public Addiction Treatment," *Addiction*, Vol. 93, No. 10, 1998, pp. 1489–1499.

McSwain, William M., Gregory B. David, John T. Crutchlow, Eric D. Gill, Bryan C. Hughes, and Erin E. Lindgren, "Complaint for Declaratory Judgment," Civil Action No. 19cv519, February 5, 2019. As of July 23, 2019: https://int.nyt.com/data/documenthelper/ 599-safehouse-complaint-final-2-5/21322f5c4bd55684f7d8/optimized/ full.pdf#page=1

"Médico búlgaro, exmilitar, Kulkin tenía, en un cuartito de Mexicali, laboratorio 'AAA' de fentanilo," *Sin Embargo*, September 18, 2018.

Midgette, Gregory, Steven Davenport, Jonathan P. Caulkins, and Beau Kilmer, *What America's Users Spend on Illegal Drugs, 2006–2016*, Santa Monica, Calif.: RAND Corporation, RR-3140-ONDCP, 2019. As of August 20, 2019: https://www.rand.org/pubs/research_reports/RR3140.html

Miller, Adam, and Nicole Ireland, "2,000% Rise in Street Drug Samples Testing Positive for Fentanyl," CBC News, November 9, 2017. As of July 11, 2019: https://www.cbc.ca/news/health/ shocking-rise-of-fentanyl-in-seized-street-drugs-1.4393906

Moore, Mark Harrison, *Buy and Bust: The Effective Regulation of an Illicit Market in Heroin*, Lexington, Mass.: Lexington Books, 1977.

Moshin, Maryam, "What Is ePacket?" *Oberlo blog*, December 5, 2018. As of July 23, 2019: https://www.oberlo.com/blog/what-is-epacket-delivery

Mounteney, Jane, Michael Evans-Brown, and Isabelle Giraudon, *Fentanyl in Europe: EMCDDA Trendspotter Study*, Lisbon, Portugal: European Monitoring Centre for Drugs and Drug Addiction, 2012.

Mounteney, Jane, Isabelle Giraudon, Gleb Denissov, and Paul Griffiths, "Fentanyls: Are We Missing the Signs? Highly Potent and on the Rise in Europe," *International Journal on Drug Policy*, Vol. 26, No. 7, 2015, pp. 626–631.

Moyer, Stephen T., Jessie Liu, and Thomas H. Carr, *2017 Annual Report for the Washington/Baltimore HIDTA*, 2018. As of July 11, 2019: http://www.hidta.org/wp-content/uploads/2018/06/ WBHIDTA-2017-Annual-Report.pdf

Musto, David F., *The American Disease: Origins of Narcotic Control*, New York: Oxford University Press, 1999.

Musto, David F., Pamela Korsmeyer, and Thomas W. Maulucci, Jr., *One Hundred Years of Heroin*, Westport, Conn.: Greenwood, 2002.

Nagin, Daniel S., "Deterrence in the Twenty-First Century," *Crime and Justice*, Vol. 42, No. 1, 2013, pp. 199–263.

National Academies of Sciences, *Pain Management and the Opioid Epidemic: Balancing Societal and Individual Benefits and Risks of Prescription Opioid Use*, Washington, D.C.: National Academies Press, 2017.

Natusch, Douglas, "Equianalgesic Doses of Opioids—Their Use in Clinical Practice," *British Journal of Pain*, Vol. 6, No. 1, 2012, pp. 43–46.

Nesser, Petter, and Anne Stenersen, "The Modus Operandi of Jihadi Terrorists in Europe," *Perspectives on Terrorism*, Vol. 8, No. 6, 2014.

Neubig, Richard R., Michael Spedding, Terry Kenakin, and Arthur Christopoulos, "International Union of Pharmacology Committee on Receptor Nomenclature and Drug Classification. XXXVIII. Update on Terms and Symbols in Quantitative Pharmacology," *Pharmacological Reviews*, Vol. 55, No. 4, 2003, pp. 597–606.

Noller, Geoffrey E., Chris M. Frampton, and Berra Yazar-Klosinski, "Ibogaine Treatment Outcomes for Opioid Dependence from a Twelve-Month Follow-Up Observational Study," *American Journal of Drug and Alcohol Abuse*, Vol. 44, No. 1, 2018, pp. 37–46.

Noor, André, Nicola Singleton, and Eleni Kalamara, *Estimating the Size of the Main Illicit Retail Drug Markets in Europe*, Luxembourg: European Monitoring Centre for Drugs and Drug Addiction, October 2018. As of July 11, 2019: http://www.emcdda.europa.eu/system/files/publications/3096/ Estimating%20the%20size%20of%20main%20drug%20markets.pdf

North American Syringe Exchange Network, homepage, undated. As of July 23, 2019: https://www.nasen.org/

O'Connor, Sean, *Meth Precursor Chemicals from China: Implications for the United States*, Washington, D.C.: U.S.-China Economic and Security Review Commission, July 18, 2016. As of July 11, 2019: https://www.uscc.gov/sites/default/files/Research/ Staff%20Report_PrecursorChemicalReport%20071816_0.pdf

O'Connor, Sean, *Fentanyl: China's Deadly Export to the United States*, Washington, D.C.: U.S.-China Economic and Security Review Commission, February 1, 2017. As of July 11, 2019: https://www.uscc.gov/sites/default/files/Research/USCC%20Staff%20Report_ Fentanyl-China%E2%80%99s%20Deadly%20Export%20to%20the%20 United%20States020117.pdf

Office of National Drug Control Policy, *National Drug Control Strategy: Data Supplement 2016*, Washington, D.C.: The White House, 2016. As of July 23, 2019: https://obamawhitehouse.archives.gov/sites/default/files/ondcp/ policy-and-research/2016_ndcs_data_supplement_20170110.pdf

Office of National Drug Control Policy, "Response to Questions Concerning Fentanyl," March 29, 2017. As of July 11, 2019; https://archives-energycommerce.house.gov/sites/ republicans.energycommerce.house.gov/files/documents/ 20170329ONDCP_Response.pdf

Office of National Drug Control Policy, "New Annual Data Released by White House Drug Policy Office Shows Record High Poppy Cultivation and Potential Heroin Production in Mexico," Washington, D.C.: The White House, July 20, 2018. As of July 11, 2019: https://www.whitehouse.gov/briefings-statements/new-annual-data-released-white-house-drug-policy-office-shows-record-high-poppy-cultivation-potential-heroin-production-mexico/

Ojanperä, Ilkka, Merja Gergov, Milana Liiv, Aime Riikoja, and Erkki Vuori, "An Epidemic of Fatal 3-Methylfentanyl Poisoning in Estonia," *International Journal of Legal Medicine*, Vol. 122, No. 5, 2008, pp. 395–400.

Ollgren, Jukka, Martta Forsell, Vili Varjonen, Hannu Alho, Henrikki Brummer-Korvenkontio, Heini Kainulainen, Karoliina Karjalainen, Elina Kotovirta, Airi Partanen, Sanna Rönkä, Timo Seppälä, and Ari Virtanen, "Amfetamiinien ja opioidien ongelmakäytön yleisyys Suomessa 2012," *Yhteiskuntapolitiikka*, Vol. 79, No. 5, 2014, pp. 513–523.

Omphroy, Lisa R., "3 Arrested in First S.D. Seizure of Synthetic Heroin Lab: Narcotics: The Drug, Fentanyl, Is Described as 60 Times More Potent Than Morphine and with a Possible Street Value of $100 Million per Pure Pound," *Los Angeles Times*, January 3, 1992. As of July 11, 2019: https://www.latimes.com/archives/la-xpm-1992-01-03-me-5574-story.html

ONDCP—*See* Office of National Drug Control Policy.

"Opium Prices Plummet, Narcos Turn to Mining and Farmers Left in Poverty," *Mexico News Daily*, December 28, 2018. As of July 11, 2019: https://mexiconewsdaily.com/news/opium-prices-plummet/

Oviedo-Joekes, Eugenia, Daphne Guh, Suzanne Brissette, Kirsten Marchand, Scott MacDonald, Kurt Lock, Scott Harrison, Amin Janmohamed, Aslam H. Anis, Michael Krausz, David C. Marsh, and Martin T. Schechter, "Hydromorphone Compared with Diacetylmorphine for Long-Term Opioid Dependence: A Randomized Clinical Trial," *JAMA Psychiatry*, Vol. 73, No. 5, 2016, pp. 447–455.

Oviedo-Joekes, Eugenia, Daphne Guh, Suzanne Brissette, David C. Marsh, Bohdan Nosyk, Michael Krausz, Aslam Anis, and Martin T. Schechter, "Double-Blind Injectable Hydromorphone Versus Diacetylmorphine for the Treatment of Opioid Dependence: A Pilot Study," *Journal of Substance Abuse Treatment*, Vol. 38, No. 4, 2010, pp. 408–411.

Paoli, Letizia, Victoria A. Greenfield, and Peter Reuter, *The World Heroin Market: Can Supply Be Cut?* Oxford, United Kingdom: Oxford University Press, 2009.

Pardo, Bryce, *Evolution of the U.S. Overdose Crisis: Understanding China's Role in the Production and Supply*, Santa Monica, Calif.: RAND Corporation, CT-497, 2018. As of July 11, 2019:
https://www.rand.org/pubs/testimonies/CT497.html

Pardo, Bryce, Jonathan P. Caulkins, and Beau Kilmer, *Assessing the Evidence on Supervised Drug Consumption Sites*, Santa Monica, Calif.: RAND Corporation, WR-1261-RC, 2018. As of July 23, 2019:
https://www.rand.org/pubs/working_papers/WR1261.html

Pardo, Bryce, Jonathan P. Caulkins, Beau Kilmer, Rosalie Liccardo Pacula, Peter Reuter, and Bradley D. Stein, *The Synthetic Opioid Surge in the United States: Insights from Mortality and Seizure Data*, Santa Monica, Calif.: RAND Corporation, RR-3116-RC, 2019. As of August 13, 2019:
https://www.rand.org/pubs/research_reports/RR3116.html

Pardo, Bryce, Lois M. Davis, and Melinda Moore, *Characterization of the Synthetic Opioid Threat Profile to Inform Inspection and Detection Solutions*, Santa Monica, Calif.: RAND Corporation, RR-2969-DHS, forthcoming.

Pardo, Bryce, Beau Kilmer, and Wenjing Huang, *Contemporary Asian Drug Policy: Insights and Opportunities for Change*, Santa Monica, Calif.: RAND Corporation, RR-2733-RC, 2019. As of July 11, 2019:
https://www.rand.org/pubs/research_reports/RR2733.html

Pardo, Bryce, and Peter Reuter, "Facing Fentanyl: Should the USA Consider Trialling Prescription Heroin?" *The Lancet Psychiatry*, Vol. 5, No. 8, 2018, pp. 613–615.

Park, Ju Nyeong, Susan G. Sherman, Saba Rouhani, Kenneth B. Morales, Michelle McKenzie, Sean T. Allen, Brandon D. L. Marshall, and Traci C. Green, "Willingness to Use Safe Consumption Spaces Among Opioid Users at High Risk of Fentanyl Overdose in Baltimore, Providence, and Boston," *Journal of Urban Health*, Vol. 96, No. 3, 2019, pp. 353–366.

Parker, Chris, "Painkiller-Laced Heroin a Fatal Attraction," *The Morning Call*, August 13, 2006. As of July 11, 2019:
https://www.mcall.com/news/mc-xpm-2006-08-13-3685264-story.html

Partanen, Airi, Hannu Alho, Martta Forsell, Elina Kotovirta, Kristiina Kuuari, Niklas Mäkelä, Sanna Rönkä, Jani Selin, and Helena Vorma, "Opioidikorvaushoito on laajentunut ja monimuotoistunut," *Suomen lääkärilehti*, Vol. 72, 2017, pp. 2981–2985.

Peiper, Nicholas C., Sarah Duhart Clarke, Louise B. Vincent, Dan Ciccarone, Alex H. Kral, and Jon E. Zibbell, "Fentanyl Test Strips as an Opioid Overdose Prevention Strategy: Findings from a Syringe Services Program in the Southeastern United States," *International Journal of Drug Policy*, Vol. 63, 2019, pp. 122–128.

"PGR Asegura Supuesto Laboratorio de Fentanilo en CDMX," *El Financiero*, December 12, 2018. As of July 11, 2019:
https://www.elfinanciero.com.mx/nacional/
pgr-asegura-laboratorio-con-elementos-para-produccion-de-fentanilo-en-cdmx

Pickard, Leonard, *Pharmacoepidemiology of a Novel Synthetic Opioid and DEA Enforcement Strategy*, Cambridge, Mass.: Harvard University, undated.

Pickard, Leonard, "Presentation to the Fellows of the Interfaculty Initiative on Drug Addictions," Harvard Faculty Club, Cambridge, Mass., 1996.

Polisen, *Swedish National Threat Assessment on Fentanyl Analogues and Other Synthetic Opioids*, Stockholm: Swedish Police Authority, 2018. As of July 11, 2019:
https://polisen.se/siteassets/dokument/
ovriga_rapporter/fentanyl-analogues-report-english.pdf

Pollack, Harold A., and Peter Reuter, "Does Tougher Enforcement Make Drugs More Expensive?" *Addiction*, Vol. 109, No. 12, 2014, pp. 1959–1966.

Pollini, Robin A., Lisa McCall, Shruti H. Mehta, David D. Celentano, David Vlahov, and Steffanie A. Strathdee, "Response to Overdose Among Injection Drug Users," *American Journal of Preventive Medicine*, Vol. 31, No. 3, 2006, pp. 261–264.

La Procuraduría General de la República, "Inicia PGR Investigación por Aseguramiento de Laboratorio Clandestino en Sinaloa," November 23, 2017. As of July 11, 2019:
http://www.miradoroaxacanoticias.com/2017/11/23/
inicia-pgr-investigacion-por-aseguramiento-de-laboratorio-clandestino-en-sinaloa/

Province of British Columbia, Public Safety and Solicitor General, "Pill Press Regulations Tackle Manufacturing of Illicit Drugs," news release, December 14, 2018. As of July 11, 2019:
https://news.gov.bc.ca/releases/2018PSSG0094-002411

Quinones, Sam, *Dreamland: The True Tale of America's Opiate Epidemic*, New York: Bloomsbury Press, 2015.

Quintana, Pol, Mireia Ventura, Marc Grifell, Alvaro Palma, Liliana Galindo, Iván Fornís, Cristina Gil, Xoán Carbón, Fernando Caudevilla, Magí Farré, and Marta Torrens, "The Hidden Web and the Fentanyl Problem: Detection of Ocfentanil as an Adulterant in Heroin," *International Journal of Drug Policy*, Vol. 40, 2017, pp. 78–83.

Raben, Dorthe, Stine Finne Jakobsen, Fumiyo Nakagawa, Nina Friis Møller, Jens Lundgren, and Emilis Subata, *HIV/AIDS Treatment and Care in Estonia: Evaluation Report*, Copenhagen, Denmark: WHO Regional Office for Europe, June 2014. As of July 11, 2019: http://www.euro.who.int/__data/assets/pdf_file/0008/255671/ HIVAIDS-treatment-and-care-in-Estonia.pdf?ua=1

Reichle, Claus W., Gene M. Smith, Joachim S. Gravenstein, Spyros G. Macris, and Henry K. Beecher, "Comparative Analgesic Potency of Heroin and Morphine in Postoperative Patients," *Journal of Pharmacology and Experimental Therapeutics*, Vol. 136, No. 1, 1962, pp. 43–46.

Reuter, Peter, "Seizures of Drugs," in Rosalyn Carson-DeWitt, Kathleen M. Carroll, Jeffrey Fagan, Henry R. Kranzler, and Michael J. Kuhar, eds., *Encyclopedia of Drugs and Alcohol*, New York: MacMillan, 1995.

Reuter, Peter, and Jonathan P. Caulkins, "Illegal 'Lemons': Price Dispersion in Cocaine and Heroin Markets," *Bulletin on Narcotics*, Vol. 56, No. 1-2, 2004, pp. 141–165.

Reuter, Peter, and John Haaga, *The Organization of High-Level Drug Markets: An Exploratory Study*, Santa Monica, Calif.: RAND Corporation, N-2830-NIJ, 1989. As of July 11, 2019: https://www.rand.org/pubs/notes/N2830.html

Reuter, Peter, Robert J. MacCoun, Patrick Murphy, Allan Abrahamse, and Barbara Simon, *Money from Crime: A Study of the Economics of Drug Dealing in Washington, D.C.*, Santa Monica, Calif.: RAND Corporation, R-3894-RF, 1990. As of July 11, 2019: https://www.rand.org/pubs/reports/R3894.html

Reuter, Peter, and Bryce Pardo, "New Psychoactive Substances: Are There Any Good Options for Regulating New Psychoactive Substances?" *International Journal of Drug Policy*, Vol. 40, 2017. pp. 117–122.

Rosenstein, Rod J., "Opinion: Fight Drug Abuse, Don't Subsidize It," *New York Times*, August 27, 2018. As of July 23, 2019: https://www.nytimes.com/2018/08/27/opinion/opioids-heroin-injection-sites.html

Rothberg, Rachel L., and Kate Stith, " Fentanyl: A Whole New World?" *Journal of Law, Medicine and Ethics*, Vol. 46, No. 2, 2018, pp. 314–324.

Rouhani, Saba, Ju Nyeong Park, Kenneth B. Morales, Traci C. Green, and Susan G. Sherman, "Harm Reduction Measures Employed by People Using Opioids with Suspected Fentanyl Exposure in Boston, Baltimore, and Providence," *Harm Reduction Journal*, Vol. 16, No. 1, 2019, p. 39.

Ruhm, Christopher J., "Corrected U.S. Opioid-Involved Drug Poisoning Deaths and Mortality Rates, 1999–2015," *Addiction*, Vol. 113, No. 7, 2018, pp. 1339–1344.

SAMHSA—*See* Substance Abuse and Mental Health Services Administration.

Schaefer, Jim, and Joe Swickard, "A Deadly Path Fentanyl-Laced Heroin Left Fatalities Nationwide," *Lowell Sun*, July 1, 2007.

Schoenherr, Tobias, and Cheri Speier-Pero, "Data Science, Predictive Analytics, and Big Data in Supply Chain Management: Current State and Future Potential," *Journal of Business Logistics*, Vol. 36, No. 1, 2015, pp. 120–132.

Scholl, Lawrence, Puja Seth, Mbabazi Kariisa, Nana Wilson, and Grant Baldwin, "Drug and Opioid-Involved Overdose Deaths—United States, 2013–2017," *Morbidity and Mortality Weekly Report*, Vol. 67, No. 5152, 2018, pp. 1419–1427.

Secretariat of the Interior, "Diario Oficial de la Federación," Mexico City, July 18, 2017. As of July 23, 2019:
http://dof.gob.mx/nota_detalle.php?codigo=5490562&fecha=18/07/2017

Selin, Jani, Pekka Hakkarainen, Airi Partanen, Tuukka Tammi, and Christoffer Tigerstedt, "From Political Controversy to a Technical Problem? Fifteen Years of Opioid Substitution Treatment in Finland," *International Journal of Drug Policy*, Vol. 24, No. 6, 2013, pp. e66–e72.

Sherman, Susan G., Kenneth B. Morales, Ju Nyeong Park, Michelle McKenzie, Brandon D. L. Marshall, and Traci Craing Green, "Acceptability of Implementing Community-Based Drug Checking Services for People Who Use Drugs in Three United States Cities: Baltimore, Boston and Providence," *International Journal of Drug Policy*, Vol. 68, 2018, pp. 46–53.

Shulgin, Alexander T., "Drugs of Abuse in the Future," *Clinical Toxicology*, Vol. 8, No. 4, 1975, pp. 405–456.

Siegfried, "Synthesis of Fentanyl," Rhodium Chemistry Archive webpage, undated. As of July 11, 2019:
https://erowid.org/archive/rhodium/chemistry/fentanyl.html

Silverman, Lester P., and Nancy L Spruill, "Urban Crime and the Price of Heroin," *Journal of Urban Economics*, Vol. 4, No. 1, 1977, pp. 80–103.

Simonsen, K. Wiese, H. M. E. Edvardsen, G. Thelander, I. Ojanperä, S. Thordardottir, L. V. Andersen, P. Kriikku, V. Vindenes, D. Christoffersen, G. J. M. Delaveris, and J. Frost, "Fatal Poisoning in Drug Addicts in the Nordic Countries in 2012," *Forensic Science International*, Vol. 248, 2015, pp. 172–180.

Smart, Rosanna, *Evidence on the Effectiveness of Heroin-Assisted Treatment*, Santa Monica, Calif.: RAND Corporation, WR-1263-RC, 2018. As of July 11, 2019:
https://www.rand.org/pubs/working_papers/WR1263.html

Smith, John, "US CA: Police Hit a Mother Lode in Drug Bust," *Washington Herald*, April 1, 2001.

Solimini, Renata, Simona Pichini, Roberta Pacifici, Francesco P. Busardò, and Raffaele Giorgetti, "Pharmacotoxicology of Non-Fentanyl Derived New Synthetic Opioids," *Frontiers in Pharmacology*, Vol. 9, No. 654, 2018.

Sordo, Luis, Gregorio Barrio, Maria J. Bravo, B. Iciar Indave, Louisa Degenhardt, Lucas Wiessing, Marica Ferri, and Roberto Pastor-Barriuso, "Mortality Risk During and After Opioid Substitution Treatment: Systematic Review and Meta-Analysis of Cohort Studies," *BMJ*, Vol. 357, 2017.

Special Advisory Committee on the Epidemic of Opioid Overdoses, *National Report: Apparent Opioid-Related Deaths in Canada (January 2016 to December 2018)*, Ottawa: Public Health Agency of Canada, 2019. As of July 11, 2019: https://health-infobase.canada.ca/datalab/ national-surveillance-opioid-harms-mortali

Spencer, Merianne Rose, Margaret Warner, Brighma A. Bastian, James P. Trinidad, and Holly Hedegaard, "Drug Overdose Deaths Involving Fentanyl," *National Vital Statistics Reports*, Vol. 68, No. 3, March 21, 2019.

Stanley, Theodore H., "The Fentanyl Story," *Journal of Pain*, Vol. 15, No. 12, 2014, pp. 1215–1226.

Statistics Estonia, "SD41: Direct Drug-Related Deaths by Sex and Age," data set, 2019. As of July 23, 2019: http://pxweb.tai.ee/esf/pxweb2008/Dialog/varval.asp?ma=SD41_en&ti=SD41% 3A+Direct+drug%2Drelated+deaths+by+sex+and+age+&path=../Database_en/ Population/04Deaths/&lang=1

Statistics Finland, "11ra: Key Figures on Population by Region, 1990–2018," data set, 2019. As of July 23, 2019: http://pxnet2.stat.fi/PXWeb/pxweb/en/StatFin/StatFin__vrm__vaerak/ statfin_vaerak_pxt_11ra.px/?rxid=21ccad08-912b-4480-8623-cfae4bce22d3

Statistics Sweden, "Population and Population Changes 1749–2018," data set, 2019. As of July 23, 2019: https://www.scb.se/en/finding-statistics/statistics-by-subject-area/population/ population-composition/population-statistics/pong/tables-and-graphs/ yearly-statistics--the-whole-country/population-and-population-changes/

Stevenson, Mark, "Mexico Opium Poppy Growers See Price Drop, Turn to Marijuana," AP News, June 22, 2018. As of July 11, 2019: https://apnews.com/cb4dac96eb24420697416c68ad92105e

Strang, John, Thomas Babor, Jonathan Caulkins, Benedikt Fischer, David Foxcroft, and Keith Humphreys, "Drug Policy and the Public Good: Evidence for Effective Interventions," *The Lancet*, Vol. 379, No. 9810, 2012, pp. 71–83.

Strang, John, Teodora Groshkova, Ambros Uchtenhagen, Wim van den Brink, Christian Haasen, Martin T. Schechter, Nick Lintzeris, James Bell, Alessandro Pirona, Eugenia Oviedo-Joekes, Roland Simon, and Nicola Metrebian, "Heroin on Trial: Systematic Review and Meta-Analysis of Randomised Trials of Diamorphine-Prescribing as Treatment for Refractory Heroin Addiction," *British Journal of Psychiatry*, Vol. 207, No. 1, 2015, pp. 5–14.

Substance Abuse and Mental Health Services Administration, "Using Fear Messages and Scare Tactics in Substance Abuse Prevention Efforts," November 30, 2015. As of July 23, 2019:
https://1jhpx52ed2l72zja983tp5xl-wpengine.netdna-ssl.com/wp-content/uploads/2018/04/fear-messages-prevention-efforts.pdf

Suh, Young-Ger, Kyung-Ho Cho, and Dong-Yoon Shin, "Total Synthesis of Fentanyl," *Archives of Pharmacal Research*, Vol. 21, No. 1, 1998, pp. 70–72.

Suzuki, Joji, and Saria El-Haddad, "A Review: Fentanyl and Non-Pharmaceutical Fentanyls," *Drug and Alcohol Dependence*, Vol. 171, 2017, pp. 107–116.

"Synthetic Heroin Seen as Cause in 18 Deaths," *New York Times*, December 25, 1988. As of July 11, 2019:
https://www.nytimes.com/1988/12/25/us/synthetic-heroin-seen-as-cause-in-18-deaths.html

Szalavitz, Maia, "Fentanyl Speedballs Are the Latest Disturbing Trend in America's Opioid Crisis," *Vice*, April 25, 2019. As of July 11, 2019:
https://www.vice.com/en_us/article/597bwb/fentanyl-speedballs-are-the-latest-disturbing-trend-in-americas-opioid-crisis

Tannenbaum, Melanie B., Justin Hepler, Rick S. Zimmerman, Lindsey Saul, Samantha Jacobs, Kristina Wilson, and Dolores Albarracín, "Appealing to Fear: A Meta-Analysis of Fear Appeal Effectiveness and Theories," *Psychological Bulletin*, Vol. 141, No. 6, 2015, pp. 1178–1204.

Tharp, Amy M., Ruth E. Winecker, and David C. Winston, "Fatal Intravenous Fentanyl Abuse: Four Cases Involving Extraction of Fentanyl from Transdermal Patches," *American Journal of Forensic Medicine and Pathology*, Vol. 25, No. 2, 2004, pp. 178–181.

Tragler, Gernot, Jonathan P. Caulkins, and Gustav Feichtinger, "Optimal Dynamic Allocation of Treatment and Enforcement in Illicit Drug Control," *Operations Research*, Vol. 49, No. 3, 2001, pp. 352–362.

Tupper, Kenneth W., Karen McCrae, Ian Garber, Mark Lysyshyn, and Evan Wood, "Initial Results of a Drug Checking Pilot Program to Detect Fentanyl Adulteration in a Canadian Setting," *Drug and Alcohol Dependence*, Vol. 190, 2018, pp. 242–245.

Tuusov, J., K. Vals, M. Tõnisson, A. Riikoja, G. Denissov, and M. Väli, "Fatal Poisoning in Estonia 2000–2009. Trends in Illegal Drug-Related Deaths," *Journal of Forensic and Legal Medicine*, Vol. 20, No. 1, 2013, pp. 51–56.

UNODC—*See* United Nations Office on Drugs and Crime.

United Nations Office on Drugs and Crime, *México: Monitoreo de Cultivos de Amapola 2015–2016 y 2016–2017*, Mexico City, November 2018. As of July 11, 2019:
https://www.unodc.org/documents/crop-monitoring/Mexico/
Mexico-Monitoreo-Cultivos-Amapola-2015-2017.pdf

United Nations Office on Drugs and Crime, *Global SMART Update: Understanding the Global Opioid Crisis*, Vol. 21, March 2019. As of July 11, 2019:
https://www.unodc.org/documents/scientific/Global_SMART_21_web_new.pdf

United Nations System Chief Executives Board, "Second Regular Session of 2018: Summary of Deliberations," Manhasset, New York, January 18, 2019. As of July 11, 2019:
https://www.unsceb.org/CEBPublicFiles/CEB-2018-2-SoD.pdf

U.S. Customs and Border Protection, "Combatting the Opioid Crisis: Exploiting Vulnerabilities in International Mail," testimony of Todd C. Owen, Executive Assistant Commissioner, Office of Field Operations before the U.S. Senate Committee on Homeland Security and Governmental Affairs," Washington, D.C., January 25, 2018. As of July 11, 2019:
https://www.hsgac.senate.gov/imo/media/doc/Owen%20Testimony.pdf

U.S. Customs and Border Protection, "CBP Enforcement Statistics FY 2019," webpage, March 31, 2019a. As of July 11, 2019:
https://www.cbp.gov/newsroom/stats/cbp-enforcement-statistics

U.S. Customs and Border Protection, *CBP Strategy to Combat Opioids*, Washington, D.C., 2019b. As of July 11, 2019:
https://www.cbp.gov/sites/default/files/assets/documents/2019-Mar/
CBP-Opioid-Strategy-508.pdf

U.S. Department of Justice, "Operation Darkness Falls Results in Arrest of One of the Most Prolific Dark Net Fentanyl Vendors in the World," press release, Washington, D.C., August 22, 2018. As of July 11, 2019:
https://www.justice.gov/opa/pr/operation-darkness-falls-results-arrest-one-most-prolific-dark-net-fentanyl-vendors-world

U.S. Department of Justice, National Drug Intelligence Center, "Fentanyl: Situation Report," Washington, D.C.: SR-000001, June 5, 2006. As of July 11, 2019:
https://www.justice.gov/archive/ndic/pubs11/20469/index.htm

U.S. Drug Enforcement Administration, *Annual Emerging Threat Report*, 2016a. As of July 23, 2019:
https://ndews.umd.edu/sites/ndews.umd.edu/files/
emerging-threat-report-2016-annual.pdf

U.S. Drug Enforcement Administration, *2016 National Drug Threat Assessment*, Springfield, Va., DEA-DCT-DIR-001-17, November 2016b. As of July 11, 2019:
https://www.dea.gov/sites/default/files/2018-07/
DIR-001-17_2016_NDTA_Summary.pdf

U.S. Drug Enforcement Administration, *Annual Emerging Threat Report*, 2017a. As of July 23, 2019:
https://ndews.umd.edu/sites/ndews.umd.edu/files/
dea-emerging-threat-report-2017-annual.pdf

U.S. Drug Enforcement Administration, *2017 National Drug Threat Assessment*, Springfield, Va., DEA-DCT-DIR-040-17, October 2017b. As of July 11, 2019:
https://www.dea.gov/sites/default/files/2018-07/DIR-040-17_2017-NDTA.pdf

U.S. Drug Enforcement Administration, *Annual Emerging Threat Report*, 2018a. As of July 23, 2019:
https://ndews.umd.edu/sites/ndews.umd.edu/files/
Emerging-Threat-Report-2018-Annual.pdf

U.S. Drug Enforcement Administration, *Fentanyl Signature Profiling Program 2017*, Springfield, Va., 2018b.

U.S. Drug Enforcement Administration, *The 2016 Heroin Signature Program Report*, Springfield, Va., 2018c. As of July 11, 2019:
https://www.dea.gov/sites/default/files/2018-10/Heroin%20Signature%20
Report%20FINAL.pdf

U.S. Drug Enforcement Administration, "China Announces Scheduling Controls on Two Fentanyl Precursor Chemicals," press release, January 5, 2018d. As of July 11, 2019:
https://www.dea.gov/press-releases/2018/01/05/
china-announces-scheduling-controls-two-fentanyl-precursor-chemicals

U.S. Drug Enforcement Administration, *2018 National Drug Threat Assessment*, Springfield, Va., October 2018e. As of July 11, 2019:
https://www.dea.gov/sites/default/files/2018-11/
DIR-032-18%202018%20NDTA%20final%20low%20resolution.pdf

U.S. Drug Enforcement Administration, *Fentanyl Signature Profiling Program 2018*, Springfield, Va., 2019.

U.S. Drug Enforcement Administration, National Forensic Laboratory Information System, *2017 Medical Examiner/Coroner Office Survey Report*, Springfield, Va., 2018. As of July 11, 2019:
https://www.nflis.deadiversion.usdoj.gov/DesktopModules/
ReportDownloads/Reports/NFLIS-MECSurveyReport.pdf

U.S. Drug Enforcement Administration, National Forensic Laboratory Information System, "National Forensic Laboratory Information System," homepage, April 29, 2019. As of July 11, 2019:
https://www.nflis.deadiversion.usdoj.gov/NFLISHome.aspx

USPS—*See* U.S. Postal Service.

U.S. Postal Service, "Postal Service Initiates ePacket Service with Hongkong Post," news release, April 20, 2011. As of July 11, 2019:
https://about.usps.com/news/national-releases/2011/pr11_037.htm

U.S. Postal Service, *Inbound China ePacket Costing Methodology: Audit Report*, Office of the Inspector General, MS-AR-14-002, February 25, 2014. As of July 11, 2019:
https://www.uspsoig.gov/sites/default/files/document-library-files/2015/ms-ar-14-002.pdf

U.S. Senate, Permanent Subcommittee on Investigations, Committee on Homeland Security and Governmental Affairs, *Combatting the Opioid Crisis: Exploiting Vulnerabilities in International Mail*, Washington, D.C., 2018. As of July 11, 2019:
https://www.hsgac.senate.gov/imo/media/doc/Combatting%20the%20Opioid%20Crisis%20-%20Exploiting%20Vulnerabilities%20in%20International%20Mail1.pdf

U.S. State Department, *International Narcotics Control Strategy Report*, Washington, D.C., March 2012. As of July 11, 2019:
https://www.hsdl.org/?abstract&did=702514

U.S. State Department, *International Narcotics Control Strategy Report*, Washington, D.C., 2014. As of July 11, 2019:
https://2009-2017.state.gov/j/inl/rls/nrcrpt/2014/

U.S. State Department, *International Narcotics Control Strategy Report*, Washington, D.C., 2015. As of July 11, 2019:
https://2009-2017.state.gov/j/inl/rls/nrcrpt/2015/index.htm

U.S. State Department, *International Narcotics Control Strategy Report*, Washington, D.C., 2016. As of July 11, 2019:
https://2009-2017.state.gov/j/inl/rls/nrcrpt/2016/

Uusküla, Anneli, Mait Raag, Sigrid Vorobjov, Kristi Rüütel, Alexandra Lyubimova, Olga S. Levina, and Robert Heimer, "Non-Fatal Overdoses and Related Risk Factors Among People Who Inject Drugs in St. Petersburg, Russia and Kohtla-Järve, Estonia," *BMC Public Health*, Vol. 15, No. 1, 2015.

Uusküla, A., K. Rajaleid, A. Talu, K. Abel-Ollo, and D. C. Des Jarlais, "A Decline in the Prevalence of Injecting Drug Users in Estonia, 2005–2009," *International Journal of Drug Policy*, Vol. 24, No. 4, 2013, pp. 312–318.

Valdez, Carlos A., Roald N. Leif, and Brian P. Mayer, "An Efficient, Optimized Synthesis of Fentanyl and Related Analogs," *PLOS ONE*, Vol. 9, No. 9, 2014.

van der Gouwe, Daan, Tibor M. Brunt, Margriet van Laar, and Peggy van der Pol, "Purity, Adulteration and Price of Drugs Bought On-Line Versus Off-Line in the Netherlands," *Addiction*, Vol. 112, No. 4, 2017, pp. 640–648.

Váradi, András, Travis C. Palmer, Nathan Haselton, Daniel Afonin, Joan J. Subrath, Valerie Le Rouzic, Amanda Hunkele, Gavril W. Pasternak, Gina F. Marrone, Attila Borics, and Susruta Majumdar, "Synthesis of Carfentanil Amide Opioids Using the Ugi Multicomponent Reaction," *ACS Chemical Neuroscience*, Vol. 6, No. 9, 2015, pp. 1570–1577.

Vardanyan, Ruben S., and Victor J. Hruby, "Fentanyl-Related Compounds and Derivatives: Current Status and Future Prospects for Pharmaceutical Applications," *Future Medicinal Chemistry*, Vol. 6, No. 4, 2014, pp. 385–412.

Varjonen, Vili, *Finland: Drug Situation 2014*, Tampere, Finland: National Institute for Health and Welfare, 2015. As of July 11, 2019:
http://www.emcdda.europa.eu/system/files/publications/984/Finland%20Drug%20Situation%202014.pdf

Vestal, Christine, "Federal Ban on Methadone Vans Seen as Barrier to Treatment," *Pew Charitable Trusts blog*, March 23, 2018. As of July 23, 2019:
https://www.pewtrusts.org/en/research-and-analysis/blogs/stateline/2018/03/23/federal-ban-on-methadone-vans-seen-as-barrier-to-treatment

Vestal, Christine, "Some Drug Users in Western U.S. Seek Out Deadly Fentanyl. Here's Why," *Pew Charitable Trusts blog*, January 7, 2019. As of July 23, 2019:
https://pew.org/2C2Trpp

Vuori, E., I. Ojaperä, T. Launiainen, J. Nokua, and R. L. Ojansivu, "Myrkytyskuolemien määrä on kääntynyt laskuun," *Lääkärilehti*, January 2012.

Walz, Andrew J., and Fu-Lian Hsu, "Synthesis of 4-anilinopiperidine Methyl Esters, Intermediates in the Production of Carfentanil, Sufentanil, and Remifentanil," *Tetrahedron Letters*, Vol. 55, No. 2, 2014, pp. 501–502.

Walz, Andrew J., and Fu-Lian Hsu, "An Operationally Simple Synthesis of Fentanyl Citrate," *Organic Preparations and Procedures International*, Vol. 49, No. 5, 2017, pp. 467–470.

Ward, C. F., G. C. Ward, and L. J. Saidman, "Drug Abuse in Anesthesia Training Programs: A Survey: 1970 Through 1980," *JAMA*, Vol. 250, No. 7, 1983, pp. 922–925.

Wells, Charlotte, and Sarah Jones, *Sustained Release Oral Morphine, Injectable Hydromorphone, and Prescription Diacetylmorphine for Opioid Use Disorder: Clinical and Cost Effectiveness, and Guidelines*, Ottawa: Canadian Agency for Drugs and Technologies in Health, April 13, 2017. As of July 23, 2019:
https://www.cadth.ca/sites/default/files/pdf/htis/2017/RB1083%20-%20Opioid%20Substitution%20Treatment%20Final.pdf

White House Council of Economic Advisers, *The Underestimated Cost of the Opioid Crisis*, Washington, D.C., November 2017. As of July 11, 2019:
https://www.whitehouse.gov/sites/whitehouse.gov/files/images/The%20Underestimated%20Cost%20of%20the%20Opioid%20Crisis.pdf

WHO—*See* World Health Organization.

Wilson, Chris M., and Catherine Waddams Price, "Do Consumers Switch to the Best Supplier?" *Oxford Economic Papers*, Vol. 62, No. 4, 2010, pp. 647–668.

Wilson, Daniel H., *Where's My Jetpack?: A Guide to the Amazing Science Fiction Future that Never Arrived*, New York: Bloomsbury Publishing, 2018.

Wish, Eric D., Amy S. Billing, Eleanor E. Artigiani, Zachary Dezman, Bradford Schwartz, and Jordan Pueschel, *Drug Early Warning from Re-Testing Biological Samples: Maryland Hospital Study*, Washington, D.C.: Office of National Drug Control Policy, Executive Office of the President, July 2018. As of July 11, 2019:
https://ndews.umd.edu/sites/ndews.umd.edu/files/
finalreport_cdews4_ed_maryland-hospital-study_part1.pdf

World Health Organization, "AH-7921 Critical Review Report," Expert Committee on Drug Dependence, Thirty-Sixth Meeting, Geneva, June 16–20, 2014. As of July 11, 2019:
https://www.who.int/medicines/areas/quality_safety/4_21_review.pdf

World Health Organization, "Joint United Nations Statement on Ending Discrimination in Health Care Settings," June 27, 2017. As of July 11, 2019:
https://www.unaids.org/en/resources/documents/2017/
ending-discrimination-in-health-care-settings

Yadav, Poonam, Jitendra S. Chauhan, K. Ganesan, Pradeep K. Gupta, Deepali Chauhan, and P. D. Gokulan, "Synthetic Methodology and Structure Activity Relationship Study of N-[1-(2-phenylethyl)-Piperidin-4-yl]-Propionamides," *Der Pharmacia Sinica*, Vol. 1, No. 3, 2010, pp. 126–139.

Zee, S. H., C. L. Lai, and Y. M. Wu, "Preparation of Fentanyl from Phenethylamine and Methyl Acrylate," *National Science Council Monthly* [K'o Hsueh Fa Chan Yueh K'an], Vol. 9, 1981, pp. 387–397.

Zee, Sheng-Hsu, and Wan-Kung Wang, "A New Process for the Synthesis of Fentanyl," *Journal of the Chinese Chemical Society*, Vol. 27, No. 4, 1980, pp. 147–149.

Zong, R., D. Yin, and R. Ji, "Synthetic Studies on Potential Analgesics. II. The Synthesis of Fentanyl (author's translation)," *Acta Pharmaceutica Sinica* [Yao xue xue bao], Vol. 14, No. 6, 1979, pp. 362–367.

About the Authors

Bryce Pardo is an associate policy researcher at the RAND Corporation. His work focuses on drug policy with a particular interest in the areas of cannabis regulation, opioid control, and new psychoactive substance markets. He has more than ten years of experience working with national, state, and local governments in crime and drug policy. Pardo holds a Ph.D. in public policy.

Jirka Taylor is a senior policy analyst at the RAND Corporation. His research interests include licit and illicit drug markets, community safety, and social and health policy interventions. Taylor holds an M.Phil. in international relations and an M.A. in American Studies.

Jonathan P. Caulkins is the H. Guyford Stever Professor of Operations Research and Public Policy at Heinz College at Carnegie Mellon University and an adjunct operations researcher at the RAND Corporation. His research focuses on modeling the effectiveness of interventions related to drugs, crime, violence, delinquency, and prevention. Caulkins holds a Ph.D. in operations research.

Beau Kilmer is the director of the RAND Drug Policy Research Center and a senior policy researcher at the RAND Corporation. His research lies at the intersection of public health and public safety, with a special emphasis on crime control, substance use, illicit markets, and public policy. Some of his current projects include analyzing the consequences of cannabis legalization; measuring the effect of 24/7 Sobriety programs on impaired driving, domestic violence, and mortality; and assessing the evidence on and arguments made about heroin-assisted treatment and supervised consumption sites. Kilmer holds a Ph.D. in public policy.

Peter Reuter is a professor in both the School of Public Policy and the Department of Criminology at the University of Maryland and an adjunct economist at the RAND Corporation. He founded the RAND Drug Policy Research Center in 1989 and was the recipient of the 2019 Stockholm Prize in Criminology. Since 1985, his research has focused mainly on alternative drug policies in the United States and Western Europe. Reuter holds a Ph.D. in economics.

Bradley D. Stein is a senior physician policy researcher at the RAND Corporation and an adjunct associate professor of psychiatry at the University of Pittsburgh. He is a health services and policy researcher with clinical experience working with children and adults with mental health and substance use disorders, and his research focuses on understanding and improving care for individuals with mental health and substance use disorders. Stein holds a Ph.D. in health policy and administration.